From Object to Icon presents the spi... raphy, contrasted with the very demanding path o... and become icons of Christ. It does this from a perspective deeply grounded in Orthodox wisdom, and without sensationalistic stories, egotistical oversharing, culture-war tub-thumping, or trivializing bits of pop culture. The book's topic deserved gravity and wisdom, and for that purpose Andrew Williams has been blessed to be a channel of God's grace.

—Khouria Frederica Mathewes-Green, author

From Object to Icon is a treasury of spiritual medicine, not only for those in the grips of addiction or attraction to pornography but for every person who lives in a culture distorted by its power. Williams defines and explains the difference between icons and idols, veneration and objectification, masks and veils, and shame and guilt, and he teaches us how to see pornography in the light of iconography and to view the world as "an icon God draws in creation." He fleshes out wisdom from earlier works by St. John of Damascus (*On the Divine Images*), St. John Climacus (*The Ladder*), Archimandrite Vasileios (*Hymn of Entry*), Fr. Pavel Florensky (*Iconostasis*), and others. I especially loved his chapter on St. Mary of Egypt—my patron saint and the object of my first novel, *Cherry Bomb*—whose life is dramatically changed when she turns her bodily and spiritual eyes on an icon of the Mother of God in Jerusalem. As we learn to allow our true selves to be seen and known through Confession and Communion, may we discover, as Williams says, that every person is an icon showing forth the image of God.

—Susan Cushman, author of *Pilgrim Interrupted, Cherry Bomb*, and "Icons Will Save the World" (*First Things*, 2007)

Andrew Williams and I became close friends and conversation partners during his days as a student here at the Holy Cross Greek Orthodox School of Theology. At that time, he was already working through the ideas that would become *From Object to Icon*. In this book, Andrew reaches out his hand to a world which, when it has not forgotten God entirely, has often forgotten how to worship Him in the ways that will lead it to freedom and integrity. I pray that for those drawn to read it, *From Object to Icon* becomes a key step in their growing closer to Christ.

—Timothy G. Patitsas, author, *The Ethics of Beauty*

"The Word became flesh and dwelt among us" (John 1:14). Saint John declares that from the beginning God intended body and soul to be in intimate relationship with one another in and through Him and the Holy Spirit.

This is a rich book—comprehensive, clearly written, and offering illuminating reflections on how the *masks, veils,* and *images* we wear can both obscure and reveal God, ourselves, and one another. No words are wasted. The author is intimately familiar with the 3D landscape of spiritual and psychological struggle that occurs between the monological pursuits of soul-deadening lust in contrast to the self-offering dialogue of love between persons infused by the joy of divine Eros. Many books already exist in the psychological literature on pornography addiction. What makes this book unique and what I most appreciate is how the author deftly explores the Orthodox Christian approach to the icon by juxtaposing it with its anti-icon, pornography, in order to reveal the way to communion between persons.

Contemporary society, increasingly dominated by virtual reality, combined with a diminishing sensitivity to contemplative presence, lacks the forbearance necessary to encounter others genuinely and wholly beyond the surface. Pornography's exponential growth and use in recent decades is a contributing factor to this developmental arrest of our capacity for intimacy with others and our diminished responsiveness to Divine Grace. But its increase is also a result of this loss and the increasing depersonalization of our lives. The author succeeds in surfacing new insights that encourage motivation to struggle to gain freedom from the shallow satisfactions of lust in pursuit of the beauty and centrality of divine Eros, which emerges from our willingness to bear the reality of one another in authentic relationship. We discover ourselves and one another anew through embracing the ascetical burden of the boundaries of love that protect the joy of authentic communion. I plan to recommend it heartily. Don't miss it!

—Fr. Stephen Muse, PhD, LMFT, pastoral psychotherapist and author of *Treasure in Earthen Vessels: Prayer and the Embodied Life, Being Bread,* and *When Hearts Become Flame*

Pornography has become the moral and psychological pandemic of the postmodern era. This digital plague contaminates human relationships by training people to be violent, revitalizing sexism, and promoting a consumptive approach of human persons. It also distorts sexuality by favoring control over participation and human scanning over deep sharing, and it manufactures female sexuality toward the male one. It is a serious lack that scientific associations of mental-health clinicians have not yet shaped a coalition against pornography. We are grateful to Andrew Williams, as his spiritual view is more than welcome. Sexuality has to be restored to a sacred initiation into the mystery of Divine Economy in which personhood is cultivated, elevated, and sanctified. Juxtaposing carnal images with icons is a fertile path because it pays tribute to our creation "in His image." In Greek we say "in His icon"; it is the same word, which makes this incredible gift sound more vivid.

—Rev. Vasileios Thermos, MD, PhD, psychiatrist for children and adolescents, and professor at the Ecclesiastical Academy of Athens, Greece

As a parish priest, I am always looking for tools to help the faithful apply the wisdom of the Faith to their real lives. Making disciples of Jesus is more than making converts, and Andrew's work will help your people to apply the real wisdom of the Incarnation and the iconographic nature of Orthodoxy to tame the passions that enslave us. With the epidemic of the indulgence of fantasy and delusion in our society that has fallen for the dead-end trap of narcissism, this helpful work will give us a path out of that slavery and into the Freedom won for us in Jesus Christ. Every parish priest and parish bookstore needs this tool.

—Fr. Barnabas Powell, parish priest at Sts. Raphael, Nicholas, and Irene Greek Orthodox Church in Cumming, Georgia, and founder of Faith Encouraged Ministries

From Object to
ICON

*The Struggle for Spiritual Vision in
a Pornographic World*

ANDREW WILLIAMS

ANCIENT FAITH PUBLISHING
CHESTERTON, INDIANA

From Object to Icon: The Struggle for Spiritual Vision in a Pornographic World

Copyright © 2023 Andrew Williams

Published by:
Ancient Faith Publishing
A Division of Ancient Faith Ministries
1050 Broadway, Suite 14
Chesterton, IN 46304

Cover image: *Adam and Eve*, Lucas Cranach the Elder. Copyright © The Samuel Courtauld Trust, The Courtauld Gallery, London.

Cover detail: The Great Panagia (Our Lady of the Sign) from the Saviour Minster in Yaroslavl, Russia.

ISBN: 978-1-955890-35-9

Library of Congress Control Number: 2023937799

Printed in the United States of America

Table of Contents

Acknowledgements

THIS BOOK HAS HAD A long gestation. The first thank-you goes to Fr. John Breck, though I have not met him, for a phrase he used in his book *The Sacred Gift of Life*, in which he describes pornography as *demonic iconography*—a phrase which stuck in my mind and started to germinate.

Thanks to many of the faculty at Holy Cross for encouraging and tolerating my interests and explorations, and particularly to Fr. Tom Fitzgerald for offering an open enough assignment back in 2008 for me to fit this topic in for my initial exploration, and to Fr. Gregory Mathewes-Green, Fr. George Morelli, and Susan Cushman for agreeing to be interviewed for that assignment. Thanks to Fr. George Dragas and Fr. Emmanuel Clapsis for supervising projects on related topics, to Dr. Evie Zachariades-Holmberg for providing me with the necessary facility in Greek to research any of these topics properly, and to Fr. Eugen Pentiuc for demonstrating daily the depth of riches a true facility in biblical and liturgical languages can yield. Additional thanks to Fr. George for being an encyclopedic source of knowledge and references, and also to the late and much missed Fr. Matthew Baker for his ability to recommend exactly the right reading for any topic. Thanks to Dr. Philip Mamalakis in particular for all of the encouragement and for the patience he has needed over the years, and also, along with Dr. Tim Patitsas and Georgia Williams, for the discussions on related matters while I was putting together the *Finding the Freedom to Live* manual. Thanks to the late and much missed Metropolitan Kallistos for blessing me to attend Holy Cross in the first place and thereby allowing all of this necessary study to happen.

Thanks to all those at Ancient Faith for their encouragement (and persistence) in getting me to write this, especially John Maddex, Katherine Hyde, and most importantly Marci Rae Johnson whose boundless patience with my various quirks made this book readable. Thanks also to others who read and advised on extracts and drafts at various stages of the process, most particularly Grainne Archer and Marchelle Brain. Thanks to all the family and friends who have put up with all of my frustrations, stresses, and lack of time during the writing! And to my confessors, spiritual fathers, and spiritual brothers and sisters who constantly inspire when I am open to inspiration, and keep me plodding on when I am not.

Without all of the above, this book would not have appeared. I have benefited from the wisdom of many, though any mistakes and misunderstandings that remain are of course my own responsibility. Please communicate them to me so that they may be corrected. Glory to God in all things!

Finally, thanks to all those I have spent time with in the course of my work as a chaplain and counselor; those who have trusted me enough to lower their masks and thereby invited me into a deeper encounter and relationship, teaching me more about love and life than I could ever imagine learning any other way.

Foreword

Blessed are the pure in heart,
For they shall see God.

—Matthew 5:8

D URING MY TWENTY YEARS AS a professor of pastoral care at
Holy Cross Greek Orthodox School of Theology, my work has
involved prayerful reading, studying, learning, and teaching about
how God's self-revelation to the world in Christ through the Orthodox Church invites each of us to fullness of life, healing, and salvation
in a variety of pastoral situations and with any number of particular
struggles. This is the Good News—that Christ is risen from the dead.
Sin and death no longer have dominion over us (Rom. 6). And Christ
invites each of us to find rest of soul by putting on the yoke of Christ,
for it is easy and His burden light (Matt. 11:30).

Yet in our lived experience we still encounter confusion, sin, loneliness, and enslavement to sinful desires. Following Christ seems
so difficult, if not impossible. And it's easy to look out at the world
around us and get the sense that sin reigns supreme and evil is out
of control and taking over. This is no more true than when we look
at the topic of pornography which, with the advent of technology in

general and the smartphone in particular, seems to have unstoppable destructive power to not only ensnare, particularly boys, at a young age, but to distort an entire culture, as Andrew Williams points out in chapter 2 of this book. It's easy to become scared of this darkness and tempting to think that we must fight to eradicate the darkness before it takes over everything . . . including the Light of Christ.

However, this reaction to fight against the darkness comes from a place of fear, not love. And, as Andrew discusses in the book, we don't conquer evil with fear but with love. This truth is built on the reality that the darkness cannot overtake the Light (John 1:5) and that perfect love casts out fear (1 John 4:18). So in the face of evil and darkness, and in this case, pornography, the answer is not a book about pornography per se but a book on the Light "of the knowledge of the glory of God in the face of Jesus Christ" (2 Cor. 4:6).

This book is not just about how to stop using pornography and is not just for those struggling with pornography addiction. This is a book about how to walk in the Light as Christians. This is a book about how to see what is real beyond physical appearances and how to connect to what is eternal through the material world. This is a book on seeing iconographically and sacramentally.

If you just read chapter 1, "Iconography and Life in Christ," you will see that this book is for everyone. Many of us never use pornography but live our lives hidden behind the masks that we create—images of ourselves as we would like people to see us. This is even true within the Church where it is easy to hide behind the practices of the Church, behind fasting, attending services, quoting the lives of the saints—looking like an Orthodox but never allowing our true, broken selves to be known by God and others. These are all beautiful masks, but burdensome masks that conceal, not reveal, our true selves. In many ways, our culture does not so much struggle with pornography but struggles with forsaking the fear of vulnerability—like Adam and Eve hiding from God and one another—and the prevalence of pornography is merely a symptom of that deeper disease. Secular therapists refer to this disease when they note the increase in narcissism in our culture. Andrew asks in his book, "Do I sometimes objectify what and whom I meet? Do I use created things and people for my own purposes, consciously or subconsciously? Do I close myself off in relationships out of fear and shame?" Andrew pulls back the veil on what clinicians refer to as narcissism and reveals it as the failure to venerate the other as icon of Christ.

The real rest for our souls and the lightness of Christ's yoke becomes apparent when we are able to repent, shed our masks, free ourselves from the burden of isolation, place our fear, shame, and struggles at the foot of the Cross, and venerate the image of Christ in each other.

When Andrew was a student of mine, I was struck by his clarity of sight and his depth of understanding of this revelation of God made man as we encounter Him through icon and sacrament. I also noticed his commitment to deepening his understanding of Orthodoxy as it pertains to those who struggle with some of the most difficult sins and passions. He spent his time at Holy Cross tirelessly reading, writing, praying, and repenting as he put together materials specifically designed to assist those struggling with powerful passions. The fruit of his personal journey, hours of research, and years of meeting together with me, Dr. Tim Patitsas, and others can be seen in his work as a therapist and chaplain, his program *Finding the Freedom to Live* (ftftl.org), and in this book, where he writes with deep insight and wisdom.

This book invites all of us who struggle with shame and fear, or struggle with pornography, sins, and passions, to direct our eyes toward Christ and purify our hearts that we may see God. It is the Light that overcomes the darkness. A life devoted to resisting temptation is wearisome, but a life devoted toward Christ, toward living in the Light, seeing clearly, and deepening our intimacy with God and others through the ascetic sacramental life of the Church is a path of freedom for all.

This book is essential for pastors and pastoral care providers walking with anyone lost in the confusion of sin that blinds us such that we see but do not perceive (Matt. 13:14). This is also a perfect book to study in groups for those who are interested in the healing that comes when we truly see with our eyes, hear with our ears, and understand with our hearts (Matt. 13:15). When we truly experience God's revelation of Himself to the world.

—Philip Mamalakis, Assistant Professor of Pastoral Care
Holy Cross Greek Orthodox School of Theology

Notes on the Text

Bible Quotations

Quotations from the Bible are my own translations of the Greek text, unless otherwise specified. The Greek source for the New Testament is the authorized 1904 text of the Ecumenical Patriarchate of Constantinople provided by the Greek Bible Society, which can be found at onlinechapel.goarch.org/biblegreek. The Greek source for Old Testament quotations is the Septuagint in the form provided by the Greek Orthodox Archdiocese of America and the Hellenic Bible Society. This can be found at www.septuagint.bible.

References and Bibliography

I have provided two lists at the end of this book for reference. The first contains academic articles and other items (primarily related to my study of academic research on pornography and associated phenomena), which I used in preparing part 1 of the book. The second is a book list covering general texts that I quote from and refer to throughout the book. I have provided author and page references in the footnotes, and the full details on these sources appear in the bibliography.

Pronouns: Individuals and Communion

In this book I tend to use the first person singular (I, me) to refer to the *individual* separated from communion and in slavery to the mask and to this fallen world of "the flesh." The first person plural (we, us) generally refers to how things are when we act, think, and experience ourselves as *in communion*, with an awareness of the true meaning of this world and God's creation.

A prayer of St. Simeon Metaphrastes sometimes included among the prayers provided for preparation before Communion begins, "As though I stood at thy dread judgement-seat."[1] It is a very long prayer and includes two lists of sins. The first is:

> Already in my works I have practiced fornication, adultery, arrogance, imposture, railing, blasphemy, foolish talking, drunkenness, gluttony, greediness, hate, envy, avarice, cupidity, graspingness, self-love, self-vaunting, robbery, injustice, covetousness, jealousy, slander, lawlessness.

And the second:

> For every work or evil, and every guile, and craft of Satan, corruption, instability, effeminacy, seduction, remembrance of wrong, counsel toward sin, forced laughter, and a thousand other passions beside have I not put aside from me. For with what sins have I not been corrupted?

I have been tempted to think it is inappropriate to say these things in the first person, as they do not seem, on first glance, to be true. And yet, reflecting more deeply and bearing in mind Christ's words that to be angry with my neighbor is to commit murder (Matt. 5:22) and

---

1   This translation is quoted from *A Manual of Eastern Orthodox Prayers*, 68, 69.

to look on a woman with desire is to commit adultery (Matt. 5:28), I find that I have, in fact, committed all of these, and the words of St. Simeon are true: "Every sin have I practiced, every prodigality have I set before my soul."

I can therefore always talk about sin in the first person. And really, this is the only appropriate way for me to talk about sin, as I do not see how I can speak of another's sin publicly without judgment. In contrast, when I speak about purity, true relationship, and communion, I am never alone. And since the ability to turn away from sin and return to communion is always open, and when I do so, I join myself with others both visible and invisible, then it is most appropriate to speak in the first person plural: this is a life to which we are all invited.

PART 1

Iconography and Pornography

Introduction

It is a soul-destroying industry and I got into it because I wanted mine destroyed.

— Former porn star[1]

PORNOGRAPHY HAS BECOME SUCH AN acknowledged problem in global Westernized society that there are now available myriad books, websites, support groups, and other resources aimed at helping people who have found themselves unable to control their pornography use. These include Covenant Eyes, Fight the New Drug, Strength to Fight, and, of course, twelve-step programs.[2] Such resources contain much that is helpful for all who find themselves involved with pornography, including ways of conceptualizing the

---

1   From a discussion with a former porn actor in an internet chat forum. Anonymous, "Ask a semi-retired porn star."

2   Covenant Eyes is a US business that produces apps, toolkits, programs, and e-books targeted at a mainly Christian audience. Fight the New Drug is an explicitly non-religious US nonprofit that aims to raise awareness of the negative effects of pornography based on education and research; they also supply an app/toolkit called Fortify. Strength to Fight is a Canadian campaigning group that also links to other resources. There are a variety of twelve-step programs (including some that are explicitly religious) that either focus on issues related to pornography or include pornography among other sex-related issues.

3

problem to help overcome the vicious circle of shame, practical steps such as finding accountability partners, and setting up a daily routine that helps avoid the spirals that lead down to pornography use.

Some resources also include wider discussions on the influence of pornography on society in general, particularly in terms of our understanding and expectations relating to sexuality and intimate relationships. Even those of us who might think we don't have any connection with pornography need to take a closer look. Our modern globalized society has increasingly "pornified" its media and advertising. "Sex sells" has been a catchphrase since the 1950s, and this applies as much to social media, art, and cinema as it does to advertising. None of us who live and work in such a society every day can remain untouched. We all need to be aware of what we are seeing, what we are unconsciously consuming, and how to address it and talk about it.

Pornography is a problem for us too in our daily lives as Orthodox Christians. In our churches and our families, some of us have an ongoing struggle with habitual pornography use, and some of us have already given up the struggle and accepted it as part of our lives. However, for Orthodox Christians, there are additional perspectives we can take on pornography, including, in particular, the perspective our iconographic tradition brings us. This tradition gives us a unique perspective on the nature of the image and the use of images that can cast light on the whole phenomenon and provide clues toward finding the freedom to live without the need to indulge addictive or habitual pornography use.

We also, of course, have our tradition of asceticism, which in recent times people have come to describe as Orthodox psychotherapy.[3] This tradition focuses on prayer, repentance, and purification through ongoing spiritual, mental, and physical struggle. One of the best-known aspects of asceticism is fasting. The path of the ascetics,

---

3   A book of this name by Metropolitan Hierotheos appeared in English in 1994.

largely overlooked in the West, provides a way of ordering our lives that is inimical to pornography use and teaches us how to strengthen our ability to resist these kinds of temptations. Thus, working through Orthodox classics that focus on this daily ascetic struggle, such as *The Ladder of Divine Ascent* by St. John Climacus, *Unseen Warfare* by St. Theophan the Recluse, or Ignatius Brianchaninov's *The Arena,* may be productive for all of us. Drawing on these resources, the *Finding the Freedom to Live* podcast on Ancient Faith Radio includes a series of four episodes called "Pathways out of Addiction," with accompanying materials on the website *Finding the Freedom to Live in the Image of God* (ftftl.org).

However, I contend that deeper healing for our struggles with pornography—and the debased use of imagery in general—will come only when we understand exactly what we are doing any time we look at another person, or indeed anything in God's creation—whether in their physical presence or in the presence of their image. Learning how to *be* in the presence of God in creation and how to *be* in the presence of any image of God will illuminate the contrast between that and the pornified gaze. Ultimately, we will find deep healing only in this transformation of the eye and the heart—and this is true for all of us, acknowledged "porn users" or not. Pornography affects all of us, directly or indirectly, and we have been taught the appetitive, objectifying way of seeing throughout our lives. Turning to the icon is where we all can find the grace of healing.[4]

In the following chapters we will:

- come to understand how the veneration of holy icons illuminates the nature of pornography and a materialist way of looking at the world;

---

4   "From Thine ikon we receive the grace of healing," stichera for Vespers on the Sunday of Orthodoxy. *Triodion,* 300.

- explore how and why pornography use might be considered an addiction, how the struggle arises and develops, and how an Orthodox way of life illuminates this issue and provides a context for finding freedom; and
- discover how we can pursue a life in Christ even in the context of our modern pornified and sexualized society.

This book is divided into four parts. The first part, "Iconography and Pornography," comprises two chapters. The first looks at iconography and our life in Christ, contrasting what we know about the holy use of images with the way people view and understand images in pornography, and setting the scene for considering pornography as shadows in the light of the holy images. The second examines the pervasiveness of pornography in our society, how the internet has contributed to this problem, how society reacts to the issue, and what secular research shows about the effects pornography has on the lives of those who use it.

The subsequent three parts deal with the way we view the world and each other from the different perspectives of masks (part 2), veils (part 3), and finally, faces (part 4). These parts investigate what each perspective tells us about our approach to pornographic imagery and to the icon, and what supports we have at our disposal to move from a pornified way of life into an iconographic one. In "Masks," we consider how, in our fallen world, we fail to perceive God through His creation. "Veils" describes the iconographic way of seeing the world and each other, wherein everything has a meaning beyond its superficial appearance and potentially links us to a deeper spiritual reality. And in "Faces," we look at how we prepare for a time when all the masks and veils are stripped away and we gain eyes to see the fullness of truth.

All the parts of the book show how our aim as Orthodox Christians is to think about the world, each other, and our experience of relationships *iconologically*. To do this, we use our experience of the veneration of icons as a way of understanding ourselves, our relationships, and the world as a whole. Our aim is to see the whole created world *iconographically*—to view the world as an icon God draws in creation.

This book is about the way we see—thus it focuses on the consumers of pornography and how a "pornified" way of looking at the world affects all of us. Whenever we speak about pornography, however, it is essential also to keep in mind those people (mostly women and girls, but also many men and boys) whom the investors, creators, and producers of pornography most directly exploit. Participation in the production of pornography is usually anything but a free choice. Many people are manipulated or coerced into appearing in it. Probably the best-known example of this is "revenge porn," in which people post compromising material such as explicit photos of former intimate partners on the web or social media. But coercion goes far beyond this. The pornography industry is built through taking advantage of people in vulnerable situations related to issues such as poverty and past abuse, and there is an established link between pornography and human trafficking. Organizations now fighting for the voices of these people to be heard include Exodus Cry, Trafficking Hub, and Collective Shout.

Even those who are not directly involved in the production of pornography are still implicated in this exploitation when they use it. In pornography, we as human beings take other vulnerable human beings and use their images to feed our baser appetites in a manner that precludes any real encounter with them. In iconography, conversely, we encounter human beings in their images, and through meeting them, we meet God. The saints in the icons are those who, rather than appropriating power over others, have poured themselves out for others, sharing in God's own willingness to make Himself vulnerable and pour Himself out for the life of the world. In this, their weakness and vulnerability become their strength, and God glorifies them.

In chapter 1 we will explore how God gives their images to us as a source of healing and sanctification, and as a means of uniting ourselves to the source of eternal life.

Iconography and Life in Christ

From Thine ikon we receive the grace of healing.... If we hold fast to the ikon of the Saviour whom we worship, we shall not go astray.

—Vespers for the Sunday of Orthodoxy[1]
(See color photo insert A.)

Icon as Participation and Encounter: A Veil

The icon is central to Orthodoxy. In fact, in Vespers for the Sunday of Orthodoxy, we sing that the icon is "the safeguard of the Orthodox faith."[2] The icon is central in our relationship with God. It is a source of healing and sanctification, and through it we can transcend the "things and facts of an objectivized and naturalized world,"[3] rediscover our personhood, and begin the journey into communion.

---

1   *Triodion*, 300.
2   *Triodion*, 300.
3   Dzalto, *Human Work of Art*, 56. When we talk about *facts* and *objectification*, we are speaking of creation divorced from the deeper meaning that is only available when we see it in its true relational context to the divine.

Because of the wonder of creation working together with incarnation, we are able to portray the image and likeness of God using created materials. And we know instinctively that in icons this depiction is also our active *participation*. Our interaction with the icon invites us into relationship with God and with the saints whom the icons portray, who stand in the immediate presence of God. In other words, the power of the icon lies in its ability to connect us with heaven— and as it makes heaven present to us in the image, it also makes us present to heaven. From our perspective, we look upon heaven by looking through the icon; from the reverse perspective of the icon, heaven looks upon us. And as our veneration of the icon passes to the prototype, God through His saints changes and sanctifies us. However, when we look upon the icon we do not see heaven directly; what we see is a sort of veil over heaven. Although the fullness of the vision of glory is hidden from my mortal and sinful eyes, the veil is a translucent covering that partially reveals what lies beyond.

In a broader sense, this concept of the icon as a veil reveals the nature of all creation if we learn to see the whole world iconographically. Saint Paul tells us this when he writes in Romans 1 about the image and how the image connects us to God: "What is known of God is revealed in them, for God revealed it to them. For since the creation of the world His invisible things, His eternal power and deity, have been clearly perceived in created things" (Rom. 1:19–20). Thus St. Paul is explaining that *everything in creation* is iconological. Icon + Logos = God the incarnate Word, visible to us.

Everything we can see is in reality calling us to something much deeper, and everything in creation transcends its material existence. Nothing is only what it seems to be on the surface—the surface we see is the veil over the uncreated. Everything points to deeper realities behind the veil. This is at the heart of what we are talking about when we speak of icons: we are talking about the relationship we can have with God through His creation and our participation in it.

Idol as Misdirection: Masks

Both historically and today, of course, iconoclasts (the "image break-ers" who fight against the use of icons) will not agree with the above description of icons, as they see any use of icons or material images of the spiritual or divine as idolatry. Romans 1 demonstrates to us why this view is wrong. I practice idolatry when I do not see through the veils of created things—when a veil becomes a mask, hiding instead of revealing the deeper truth, and misdirecting me from the real meaning of what I see. I practice idolatry when I see the created thing only in itself, and instead of seeing the power and glory of God in what He has created, I invest the creation itself with power. Similarly, in pornography I specifically see the flesh; I do not see through the veil of the flesh to the deeper reality. Rather than seeing a veil that reveals the ultimate source of Love, I see a mask that holds no significance beyond itself or that misdirects me away from love in truth. I do not see an image-bearer of God but rather flesh for my own satisfaction.

We can go further and say that this wrong way of seeing is actually theft. I steal from God when I take His image and separate it from its physical manifestation: I steal the image of God. I also steal from the other person when I close my eyes to the person's true ultimate signif-icance and regard them as flesh, which I manipulate for my own pur-poses. But the gold I steal turns to dust in my hands: I not only lose the relationship I am supposed to find with God—and with others—through His creation, but I find that what I have lost was what I was really seeking. It turns out that this relationship was what was really valuable and meaningful in what I took for my own pleasure.

This is all about relationship: I can go deeper into intimacy by seeing through the veils, or I can avoid intimacy by getting lost in the masks. I develop a relationship or exclude myself from it partly because of how I see, how I look at another person. My relationship with a person can go deep if I can see deeply—if I can see behind the veils of the external or physical image. But my relationship with a person cannot go deep if I refuse to see the true reality beyond what my physical senses can immediately access.

I also develop or damage a relationship according to what I give of myself: do I open the true and deep reality of myself in relationship, or do I hide it, holding it privately deep within, behind my masks? If I use pornography, I not only refuse to see beyond the surface of the other, but I also refuse to reveal or even acknowledge the deeper reality within myself. When I do this, I freeze life, I objectify: that is, I make another person an object for my own use. I fight against the true dynamic nature of life as God created it. I refuse to allow another person to be real and to transcend the physical body. This is of course a dramatic breaking of the greatest commandment: to love the Lord our God with all our hearts, all our minds, and all our souls, and to love our neighbors as ourselves. To objectify another is to refuse to love God, neighbor, and even self.

In summary, then, my refusal to see properly, to see beyond the physical material presented to me, is a theft from God, from the other, and from my own true self. It is idolatry, as I refuse to see God in His creation. In effect, it is a refusal to live, to love, to relate, and to see or accept the image of God and His love.

Image of God

How we address this refusal to see properly is not a question only for habitual or even occasional users of pornography. We are all suffering from a disease of which pornography use is a particular form. To start healing from this disease, we need to know that every encounter with every person is an encounter with the person as the image of God. As Orthodox Christians, we know something about how to treat icons with respect, but do we know how to treat the image of God in every person with respect? Those of us who have been blessed by an encounter with someone who truly sees the image of God in us will know how much that means and the transformation it can engender.

From our experience venerating icons, we can learn to view every encounter with another person as an opportunity to see and venerate the image of God. Every person is an icon showing forth the image of God; when we see an icon, we venerate it, even when it is old or damaged. Only when the icon is broken beyond repair—when the image is totally effaced—will it be taken out and thrown into the fire (John 15:6). In St. John's Gospel, only the dead vine branches are cast into the fire—those branches that are no longer attached to Christ the True Vine. In St. Matthew's Gospel, the ones cast into the fire are those who fail to see Christ, the true Image of God, in others (Matt. 25:41). If I cannot see and love Christ in another human being, the result is the same as being cut off from the source of life within myself. Loving God with all our heart, soul, and mind implies loving our neighbor as ourselves (Matt. 22:37). We cannot separate these two things.

However, no human person still living is broken beyond repair. The life-giving presence of the image of God is the reason we live; hence, however damaged the person, we can still look them in the eyes and see the image of God. And however damaged I am, any saint can look at me and see an icon of Christ. There is hope for all of us. But looking at people in this way is not easy; it may not come naturally. Because of the fallen nature of this world (and of all of us who live in it), we cannot immediately access the image of God. The likeness is impaired; it is veiled in all of us to a greater or lesser extent. But it is precisely through learning to venerate icons that we can begin to learn in this life what it means to truly see what is beyond—the fullness of life beyond the veil.

In this way the Church is the hospital where we begin to find healing for the sickness of sin that impairs our likeness to God. Saint John of Damascus illustrates this when he writes:

> Suppose I . . . walk into the spiritual hospital—that is to say, a church—with my soul choking from the prickles of thorny thoughts, and thus afflicted I see before me the brilliance of the icon. I am refreshed as if in a verdant meadow, and thus my soul is led to glorify God.[4]

The Seventh Ecumenical Council likewise connects our embrace of the icon with healing and sanctification, proclaiming, "When we embrace an icon and offer to it the veneration of honor, we share in sanctification."[5] Strengthened by the refreshment St. John of Damascus mentions, sanctified by the holy icons, and learning from our liturgical experience, we can begin to see the image of God even when it is veiled, when it is seen "in a mirror, dimly" (1 Cor. 13:12).

As we embrace the icon in love, through love we begin to approach what lies behind the veil of our fallen world. As St. Paul puts it, "When the fulfillment comes, then the partial will be of no effect. . . . Now I know in part, but then I shall recognize just as I also am recognized" (1 Cor. 13:10–12). This is the opposite of idolatry and of objectifying another; this is the fullness of interpersonal relationship, wherein we see and are truly seen, we know and are truly known. The question for each of us is: Which do I really do in everyday life—venerate or objectify? Can I learn to see a fuller reality and the ultimate significance of every person beyond what my physical senses perceive, which will enable me to move into deeper communion with God and others and into a greater fullness of life? Or will I objectify the people

---

4   From Treatise I.47. Powell, "Pneumatology," 341.
5   Sahas, *Icon and Logos*, 99.

and things I see around me, breaking within my own heart the intimate connection between God and His creation?

Desire

We read in Genesis 2:18 that, "It is not good for the person to be alone." This is one of the foundational things we know about the human person, right from the beginning. The deepest part of each of us desires to reach out of ourselves and make a connection. So, though it may sound strange to say it, the impulse to embrace the icon and the temptation to embrace pornography spring at root from the same thing: the desire to connect. This should not be a surprise, as we know that evil has no existence in its own right; it is always derived from something good: it is "good gone wrong."

All desire at its root is the desire to make a connection—to unite ourselves with something or someone else. And the desire to make a connection is in itself good. It is not only something God gave us in the beginning but something that reflects His own life in us. His desire for us is so strong that He consents to empty Himself, descend to us, take flesh, and live bodily with us (Phil. 2:5–8; John 1:1–18). Our deepest and most authentic desire is the same: to be united in soul, mind, and body with Him. This, however, cannot be experienced in its fullness until the marriage supper of the Lamb at the end of all things (Rev. 19:9), when everything we have ever desired finds fulfillment in the total and intimate union of all creation in Christ (1 Cor. 15:28) and our participation in the very life of God (2 Pet. 1:4).

The desire that drives anyone toward pornography is a worldly fact that will be transformed if we learn to venerate, to love—as we learn to be a person in communion. Through this transformation, the image of God develops into the likeness of God in us. His self-emptying can lead to our fulfillment, His descent to our ascent, His presence in this earthly life to our participation in the divine life.

"God became man so that man could become God,"[6] St. Athanasius wrote in *On the Incarnation*, and because of the Incarnation, it became possible to portray God in an icon. The Incarnation gave us this way of seeing the truth: it is in the flesh and through the flesh that we can see God.

Thus, the first question I ask myself is what worldly fact in my own life can be transformed into love and veneration? Which of my immediate desires contradict or short-circuit my deeper desires? Which are temptations aimed at something much less than love and union with God? So if I have used pornography, I ask myself why. Out of what need or desire does this temptation arise? If I have a close friend or relative who is struggling with habitual pornography use, I ask them why. What are they longing for? What are they really seeking? What need are they trying to fill?

The answers I receive to these questions always on some level come back to the desire—the need—to make a connection. To fill my emptiness. To feel that I have a real existence in the world. To reach out of this lonely body and bring myself together with another. So on the one hand, I desire relationship. But on another level, answers to these same questions also come back to the wish to short-circuit relationships. I see this particularly in answers like, "My wife doesn't fulfill my sexual needs" or "I want an easy and quick way of reaching sexual release."

So as well as seeing what iconography and pornography have in common—the deep need for connection—here we can also see the distinction between iconography and pornography. Praying with an icon is a way of opening myself to the other. It is about love, and it is about veneration. It requires that I invest myself in the relationship. It requires that I make myself vulnerable and acknowledge my vulnerability, and it shows my true face as I look into the true face of a sanctified

---

6   Athanasius, *On the Incarnation*, 54.

other. It is a means of seeing through the veil—and being seen through the veil—and making contact with God through His creation.

Pornography, on the other hand, is about opening the other to me while cutting myself off, not only from them but even from my own truer, deeper self. It is about idolatry, as I seek my meaning and ful-fillment in the creation rather than the Creator. It requires nothing of me except what I want to give, and it enables me to take power over the other without taking any of the responsibility. It enables me to hide myself, my fears, my inadequacies, and pretend they don't exist. It is putting on a mask and failing to see beyond the masks of oth-ers. It cuts off any possible link with the deeper reality beyond the psycho-physical, which means it cuts me off from God and abuses His creation.

When I stand in front of an icon, I venerate; I open myself to a transcendent Reality. Part of veneration is being seen, and the reverse perspective of the icon puts me in the frame. As I look through the icon, the sanctified other looks upon me. In this process, I give of myself and I receive from the other. When I place myself in front of pornography, I objectify or idolize; I close myself within myself; I take from the other without offering anything of myself, and I remain unseen.

But in practice, every kind of desire turns out to be part of a recip-rocal process of relating. In this sense, I am formed by my desire. Even if my desire appears to be one-sided, it is not possible to desire without to some degree opening myself to what I desire. And in doing so, I unwittingly cause myself to change. So I can ask, "What does this particular desire do to me? What kind of person am I becoming as I exercise it in this way?" Every encounter changes me, and the way I respond to my desire—particularly the way I habitually respond—shapes my soul just as it shapes the pathways in my brain.[7] It grows

---

7   See chapter 8 for more on the processes of habitual patterns and addictions.

me into a particular kind of person. My character is formed by my desires, thoughts, feelings, and actions and by the way I relate to others and to God through the internal promptings of desire. In turn, my developing character affects my desires, thoughts, feelings, and actions, and it affects how I relate to others and to God.

As this character formation plays out at the societal level, we have seen over the last few decades a "pornification" of culture as more and more people have uncritically followed their desires down the pornified "broad" path (Matt. 7:13). As pornography becomes more normalized, the images that surround all of us every day become more sexualized. This becomes a vicious circle. Following my desires changes not only me and those directly in contact with me, but also the broader world around me, and the increasingly pornified society in which I live then in turn changes my desires.

Here is one example of this: Women who marry men who have habitually used pornography tell us that their husbands expect sexual behaviors from them that make them feel uncomfortable. Why? Because if I have habitually used pornography, I am used to controlling sex and focusing it on my own pleasure. I am used to closing up myself and my own deepest needs and living in an objectified, idolized physical reality. I have no way to truly meet another person at a deep level, no way to be vulnerable, and in the end, therefore, no way to meet God.

It is important to stress that, since as human beings we are a body-mind-spirit unity, everything we do with our bodies affects our spiritual reality. Everything we do with our minds affects our spiritual reality. In the end, every act, every thought, every way we indulge our desires leads us closer either to heaven or to hell. That is, either to an eternity where we participate in the very life of God, or to an eternity where I am totally cut off from God and closed in on myself and my own pain. Our desire exists precisely to lead us to connection: to transcend this sense of being cut off from the things we need and desire. Desire is not only a gift from God but something that reflects God's very nature: again, this is the iconological nature of reality. But all that is satanic, demonic, and sinful wants to twist this desire so that it no longer points to ultimate fulfillment in union with God through His creation. Rather it becomes a desire that ultimately leads nowhere, seeing the creation as an end in itself.

But what is the starting point from which I can grow closer to God—feeling the desire but misdirecting it, or training myself not to feel the desire at all? Saint John Climacus says, "Not he who has kept his clay undefiled is pure, but he who has completely subjected his members to his soul."[8] Thus, we should not attempt to kill our desires but welcome their transformation into a full-bodied, whole-hearted desire for God.

Veneration or Objectification?

In a sense, each one of us is a pornography addict with a tendency to see God's creation as objectified flesh and not as icon. Do I venerate every person I meet as the image of God? Do I look at creation as a veil that reveals to me the contours of God Himself? Do I open myself in every encounter to receive what God offers through it? Do I, as St. Paul says, concentrate my attention on everything that is true, honorable, pure, lovely, and commendable (Phil. 4:8)?

Or do I sometimes objectify the things and people I meet? Do I use created things and people for my own purposes, consciously or subconsciously? Do I close myself off in relationships out of fear or shame? When I do, I am turning away from God. I am being unfaithful to Him, and unfaithfulness is the characteristic act of immorality. It is one of the senses of *porneia*. If I do these things, I am reading

---

8   Climacus, *Ladder*, 15:10, 105.

19

God's creation as a superficial, obscene writing—*pornography*—and not as the writing of God's image—*iconography*—that it truly is.

Once I understand that I am not cut from some totally different cloth from the porn addict, I am ready to stand alongside him or her and begin the work of turning both of us around toward the face of God. With all this in mind, we are ready to examine the phenomenon of pornography and the particular way it has taken root in our society.

CHAPTER 2

Pornography and Society

The more a man leads the carnal mode of life, the more carnal he becomes: . . . he sees flesh and matter in everything, and nowhere, nor at any time, is God before his eyes.

—Saint John of Kronstadt[1]

S O FAR I HAVE BEEN talking as if we all know what pornography is and agree on its definition. In this chapter, I will look more closely at the definition and then move out to consider the place pornography has come to have in our society—why we find it tempting, how much its use has spread, and its effect on us both personally and as a society.

What Is Pornography?

Words that have a common root with the Greek word πορνεία (*porneia*) in apostolic times related to various kinds of sexual immorality and particularly to prostitution. Words with this root are

---

1   John of Kronstadt, *My Life in Christ*, 143.

connected with unfaithfulness and idolatry. As far back as the time of Hosea the prophet, sexual unfaithfulness was tied to idolatry in the image of God's marriage to his people and his people's unfaithfulness to Him. The Greek γραφή (*graphē*) means something drawn, painted, or written. Hence the straightforward etymological meaning of the word *pornography* is "imagery or text relating to sexual immorality and unfaithfulness."

Another way of expressing this etymology which has arisen in the last ten years or so is to define pornography as "filmed prostitution."[2] Some women who have previously been involved in prostitution describe it as "paid rape" or "pay-as-you-go rape."[3] This would make pornography "filmed paid rape."

The *Oxford English Dictionary* defines pornography as "the explicit description or exhibition of sexual subjects or activity in literature, painting, films, etc., in a manner intended to stimulate erotic rather than aesthetic feelings." Most modern academic research on pornography follows the two aspects of this definition: media that are (a) sexually explicit and (b) stimulate sexual arousal. Studies often leave it up to the user to define whether or not something fits in the category of pornography, and some researchers make the point that it is hard to define pornography only by content. Since part of the definition relies on inciting sexual arousal, the context and intention of the viewer are also relevant.[4]

---

2   Perhaps the earliest popular use of this expression appears in a 2013 article by Ran Gavrieli, a sex-education activist, in the German feminist magazine *Emma*. The comparison between pornography and prostitution, however, was discussed at length in the 2000s in particular, but it goes back at least to Kathleen Barry in 1979. See Tyler, "Harms of Production."

3   Moran, *Paid For*, 113.

4   E.g., Malamuth, "Pornography," 11817; Attorney General, 228–29. In a perhaps slightly euphemistic version of the same definition, Barron and Kimmel, 162, define it as "any sexually explicit material to which access was limited, either by signs or physical structure, to adults." Many academic studies fail to define what they include as pornography, so they often leave it to the

For the purpose of this chapter, therefore, I consider the definition of *pornography* to be media relating to sexual immorality and unfaithfulness that are sexually explicit and designed to stimulate or arouse.[5] It is important to be aware that different authors use the word *pornography* in various ways, and in using this relatively limiting definition, we are not including art and media representing the human form, sexuality, or eroticism which do not relate to immorality or unfaithfulness.[6] When we go on in subsequent chapters to consider the way we look at the world in general, I will explore the limits of this definition to argue that all cases of iconoclastic vision—refusing to see the reality beyond the physical surface—are a form of unfaithfulness to God and are, in this sense, pornographic.

Some research[7] suggests that in general, a greater proportion of women use online sexualized chat, rather than image- and video-based pornography, as compared to men. This may also be true of

---

self-assessment of the participants in the research (see Mikkola, *Pornography*; Esplin, "What motives drive?").

5   This is similar to the definition of Canon 100 of the Quinisext Council of 692: "pictures . . . which attract the eye and corrupt the mind, and incite it to the enkindling of base pleasures" (NPNF-II, XIV: 407). Today, videos make up a greater proportion than pictures. Lap dancing and live sex shows are a slightly different, albeit related, category, but I am not including them here as they are not media. Cam sites lie somewhere in between (see e.g., Mikkola, *Pornography*). Whether we consider so-called "revenge porn" and recorded footage of sexual abuse as pornography in my estimation depends on context, as it may, for example, be produced as evidence in a trial, or it may be uploaded to the internet for gratification.

6   Examples of these might include sexually explicit imagery for medical or anatomical purposes, classical sculpture, nudity in art, etc. Neither sexual explicitness nor sexual arousal (which is individual or context specific) is an adequate category, and this is where the research struggles to make clear distinctions. Some research uses the expression "sexually explicit" media to adopt a neutral tone, whereas others do not see the word *pornography* itself as pejorative. Still others distinguish the negative *pornography* from a supposed positive *erotica* (for example, see Flood and Hamilton, *Youth and Pornography in Australia*).

7   E.g., Green et al., "Cybersex Addiction Patterns."

pornographic literature. We can consider all of these as forms of pornography,[8] but I will focus here on the more common understanding
of pornography as relating to visual images—in other words, mostly
photos and videos (though also cartoons, drawings, and animations).
Later in the book I will also discuss sexual and relational fantasy—
pornographic imagery in the mind.

The etymological definition puts the focus squarely on the harmful effects of pornography, whether these be physical, psychological,
or spiritual. I root my argument against pornography, therefore, in
the fact that it is intrinsically harmful to all its participants on both
sides of the screen: it is both a cause and a result of spiritual sickness,
or sin. Unlike some researchers, I do not see a meaningful distinction
in practice between "morally corrupting" and "harmful";[9] I see these
as two sides of the same coin.

Sexually explicit images date back to ancient times, but transgressive imagery designed specifically to transgress social conventions
for the purposes of sexual arousal may be a more recent phenomenon.

---

8   I exclude a consideration of online chat and pornographic literature here
    as these are slightly different categories, though they can be pornographic
    in words and can involve imagery in terms of giving rise to pornographic
    fantasies, which I will discuss later. I also do not include a specific discussion
    of cam sites, which are the most immediate form of "filmed prostitution."

9   Those who critique pornography from a secular perspective may on the one
    hand focus on the obscene or indecent nature of pornography, or on the other
    hand they may critique the concepts of obscenity and public morality and
    yet still see harm in pornography, for example because of the discriminatory,
    violent, or oppressive nature of the imagery in question. A distinction is often
    made in the US between what is seen as morally unacceptable and what is
    harmful, based on the constitutional protection of "free speech," which in
    this context has a specific legal definition (see Mikkola, *Pornography*, 99–106
    for a discussion of this). My use of "harmful" here includes harm to the self,
    not only to others, and I consider that anything that is morally corrupting is
    by definition harmful—physically, psychologically, and/or spiritually. I am
    not making any argument here for what, if anything, should be done legally
    to prohibit pornography; that is a different discussion beyond the scope of
    this book.

Some date this to the seventeenth century.[10] The eighteenth and nineteenth centuries saw the advent of mass-produced erotic literature, and the invention of photography in the mid-nineteenth century immediately resulted in sexually explicit photography. By the early twentieth century, sexually explicit films came into existence. In the mid-twentieth century, the popularity of the "pinup" photo gave birth to so-called "men's" magazines, beginning with *Playboy* in 1953. Full nudity appeared in these magazines beginning in the late 1960s, and by the 1970s, they also included sexual activity and fetishes. The 1980s saw the dramatic growth of home video, and with that came both legal and illicit pornographic videos.[11]

In the 1990s the ability to access the internet, however, marked major changes. It massively increased the availability of pornography, cut out any need for a middleman, made legislation to limit access difficult to design and enforce, democratized not only the consumption of pornography but also its production, and created access to an immediate global audience. As popular use of the internet increased, pornography increased with it, on the back of which the pornography industry (which had come into existence with the magazines), especially pornographic video, grew exponentially. Over time, perhaps due to a combination of competition and the need to maintain the level of stimulation by using ever more transgressive scenes, the content of pornography has become increasingly explicit, fetishistic, and violent.[12]

---

10 Tarrant, *The Pornography Industry*, 11.
11 Tarrant, Chapter 2.1–4.
12 This is a controversial topic in the research literature. Some recent studies claim that this is not the case, but many of these arguments are flawed for the following reasons: First of all, the change may not be significant in the short term (e.g., the last ten years or so), but it becomes much clearer when, for example, comparing pornographic imagery from the 1970s or '80s to that from the last ten years or so. Other reasons include either a selective use of videos/images or a questionable assessment of when a video or image is or

It is apparent that two key themes in pornography are power and violence. The act of consuming pornography is an act of taking power over other people through sexual desire in a way that is impossible to achieve in a real-life sexual encounter (other than by committing a serious crime). This is because the people on the screen never have the option to let their desires be known or even simply to withhold consent. It is an act which instrumentalizes or objectifies another human person or persons to satisfy one's own desire. Much of the feminist critique of pornography focuses on this—the fact that most pornography is on some level about subordination, even when it is less explicitly violent or abusive. Because the majority of porn consumers are male and the majority of those appearing in pornography are female, this is an example of male exploitation and abuse of women: of men engaging in a medium that automatically puts women under their power and control.

Outside the sexual realm, the most common use of the word *lust* is probably in the expression "lust for power." There is a strong link between sexual immorality, power, and violence. Some argue that the exercise of this power in pornography is different because it is "imaginary": the person is not really present to me, and I am not really using the actual person for my own gratification, just the image. "Imaginary," however, is not the opposite of "real." Every image, including a mental image, has its own significance, as I will discuss in a later chapter when considering the role of fantasy. It is also important to note that pornographic imagery would not have come into existence if there were no consumers. Therefore, everyone who watches a video

---

isn't counted as violent or aggressive. For example, researchers may select only the most popular videos to assess (rather than assessing how much of the content is violent) and/or may not count a video as aggressive or violent unless the person who is the object of the aggression either complains or indicates hurt or displeasure in the video (which does not take into consideration the context of the porn set and the director's power). See, for example, Bridges et al., "Aggression and Sexual Behavior"; Flood, "Pornography, violence."

or looks at an image for sexual gratification is in fact participating in the actual use/abuse of the person portrayed.

An Orthodox understanding of image should immediately preclude such arguments. What is a person if not an image of God? And yet in pornography each image of God is depersonalized or fetishized into an objectification of some aspect of their humanity—their sex, age, race or ethnicity, an aspect of their physical characteristics, their job, role, or social status. In other words, pornography is about a performance of some aspect of identity that is inhumanly elevated above the personal or interpersonal. This is true not only for the performer or the person portrayed; it is also true of the viewer. If I view pornography, I am avoiding the opportunity to engage with real relationship in favor of dehumanizing not only myself but also the object of my attentions in a relationship of nothingness that can lead nowhere. This exaggeration of objectified flesh is taken to the highest degree in so-called *hentai*, anime-style pornography, in which cartoons and animations portray stylized, exaggerated, and super-stereotyped bodies and actions, exhibiting an emphatic destruction of the personal, of the image of God, in favor of the ultimate in objectification.

Returning to the portrayal of real human beings as sexual objects, it is important to stress again that participation in the creation of online pornography is usually not entirely voluntary. The clearest examples of this are so-called "revenge porn" and videos made of occasions of sexual abuse. Pornography of these types is widely available on many pornographic websites, which don't differentiate it in any meaningful way from any other kind of pornography. However, even when the person appearing in pornography acts supposedly by choice, there is plenty of evidence of manipulative and coercive practices either used to get the performer involved in the first place, or in terms of what she or he is required to do on set.[13]

---

13   E.g., Grudzen et al., "Pathways to Health Risk" and "Comparison of Mental

What Is the Attraction?

Now that I have painted this overwhelmingly negative picture of what pornography is, we need to consider what causes anyone to want to consume it. Perhaps the most obvious answer to this is the unavailability of a real, intimate relationship and/or the fear of entering into one. However, the research identifies a number of motivations, almost exclusively self-reported by pornography users (usually selected from a predefined list of options). These include sexual pleasure, sexual curiosity, emotional distraction or suppression, stress reduction, fantasy, boredom, avoidance, self-exploration, and lack of sexual satisfaction.[14] Low self-esteem, loneliness, and social anxiety are also factors the research identifies.[15] This suggests that if I turn to pornography, I may perceive either that it will help me avoid the feelings associated with low self-esteem and loneliness, or that it will help me actually overcome these issues by filling the emptiness. There are two main themes here: my desire for connection (even if it is illusory) and my avoidance—whether I am seeking to avoid emptiness, fear, difficult emotions or relationships, or the world as a whole when it has begun to feel unmanageable.

Additionally, I may see pornography as a way to gratify sexual desire without technically cheating.[16] I could argue that there is no infidelity because I have had no physical contact with another person and/or because the relationship is imaginary (that is, not reciprocal—it only exists in the mind of the pornography user).

Health"; Javanbakht et al., "Transmission Behaviors"; Donevan, "No Longer Human." Many of the campaigning and support organizations also provide numerous personal stories of negative experiences people have had during their involvement with the pornography industry.

14   E.g., Bőthe et al., "Why do people watch." It is worth noting that in this study, men demonstrated higher scores than women on all motivations except for sexual curiosity and self-exploration.

15   Wery et al., "Problematic online sexual activities."

16   Wery et al.

Faithfulness, however, is not a technicality, and few spouses find this justification convincing. Unfaithfulness is the act of turning away. That applies regardless of what or whom we turn toward when we seek a sexual connection (even a so-called "imaginary" one) apart from our spouse.

Pornography—especially online pornography—also offers the ability to remain anonymous. The perceived need for anonymity relates largely to the experience of shame, such as that related to certain sexual desires, fantasies, or fetishes. The internet seems to provide an arena where I can indulge my desires without being seen and judged: it seems to offer the opportunity I do not easily find in real life to be shameless. This promise, however, is also illusory, as I will discuss later in the chapter.

However strong this interest in anonymity is, however, desire is always about connection, and we can see how all the things that make pornography attractive seem to offer the possibility of that connection or fulfillment. Nevertheless, all human desire is in the last analysis a desire for God and the fullness of the eternal union of all in Him. Thinking iconologically, we can describe these desires themselves as icons. Desires for what is created are icons of the greater desire for the infinite: all our physical desires are ways in which we as physical creatures can meet God through His creation. Sexual desire is a desire for physical union with another person, which itself is an icon of the fullness of the eternal union with God—when we will participate in the divine nature. This is what makes sexual temptation attractive—it is a subtle twisting of our true desire. This is why the link between sex and idolatry has been so strong since ancient times, and why the characteristic scriptural image of the relationship of God and Israel, or Christ and the Church, is one of marriage. If I channel my desire for sexual union into the dead end of pornography, it is a subversion of this connection in the same way that the worship of an idol is: it fails to see the Creator through His creation and instead sees the creation as an end in itself, which is an act of unfaithfulness to the Creator. Ultimately, this idolatry means that I form a relationship with what cannot truly live instead of with the source of life. It is this idolatrous nature of pornography that makes it soul-destroying.

Pervasiveness

Just how pervasive is pornography? While the statistics below relate specifically to sexually explicit imagery, it is important to remind ourselves again that there is no radical discontinuity between pornography and the rest of our culture. When we remember that the etymology of pornography refers to imagery about sexual immorality or unfaithfulness, it is easy to see a much broader application than that of sexually explicit imagery alone. If we think back to films and television we have enjoyed or songs we like, for example, can we say they are all free of sexual immorality and unfaithfulness?

In fact, the technological development of the internet that brings all these media to us is directly connected to pornography. Many of the early online business successes were related to the pornography industry, and pornography was also a driver of much early internet technology, especially that relating to video. This technology led to a massive increase in the use of pornography from the turn of the twenty-first century onward. Even by the mid-1990s, the majority of digital imagery available online within Usenet was pornographic.[17] By the early 2000s there were somewhere between 23 million and 60 million unique visitors to pornography websites each day, and about half of Christian pastors in the US identified internet pornography as a current struggle. Offline, almost three-quarters of

---

17 Usenet is an online discussion system based on "newsgroups" on the internet, which has been in existence since 1980, predating the existence of the World Wide Web. See Rimm, "Marketing Pornography."

in-room movie revenues in hotels were from pornographic films.[18] By the 2010s, major hotel chains began to drop pornographic films from their in-room systems, most likely primarily because of falling revenues due to the competition from free pornography available on smartphones.[19] Pornography is also easily accessible on most forms of social media and through web searches.[20]

In 2019, one major pornography site alone attracted around 115 million visits per day, which was more visits than Netflix or Zoom received.[21] Visitors stayed for an average of over ten minutes each visit. If you wanted to watch just the new videos posted on that site alone in 2019, it would take you more than 150 years of continuous viewing (plus any sleeping hours you might need).[22]

Back in 2005, a US national survey revealed that a quarter of men and 4 percent of women reported viewing pornography online within the last month. By 2020, as many as nine out of every ten men and six out of ten women in the US had accessed pornography within the previous month.[23] An Australian survey in 2017 of young people aged 15–29 found that practically all the boys and men and most of the girls and women reported viewing pornography.[24]

---

18 Statistics from Coleman, "Porn in the USA," and Paul, *Pornified*, 20, 55.
19 E.g., Harpaz, "Hyatt hotels." In the same period, many ISPs dropped access to Usenet, ostensibly related to child pornography concerns, but some speculate that the primary motivation was to reduce costs.
20 For example, Twitter expressly permits pornography, with the only safeguard being a request that users mark such content as "sensitive" (Twitter, 2021). Other forms of social media have varying rules, but in practice there is limited enforcement of any restrictions, even on non-consensual explicit imagery. See for example Henry and Witt, "Governing Image-Based Sexual Abuse." Google has a SafeSearch option, but it is off by default, and even if on, it is easy to disable.
21 Khalili, "most popular websites."
22 Published figures from the site.
23 Mirzaei, "Hijab Pornography."
24 Lim et al., "Young Australians'." They found 257 of 258 young men surveyed reported viewing pornography.

Statistics about the number of children and young people accessing online pornography vary, but it is clear that there is extensive teen usage and that a majority of children (particularly boys) have been exposed either accidentally or on purpose to internet pornography before the age of thirteen. Surveys suggest that parents are not aware of this. A UK survey from 2020 found that three-quarters of parents of children aged eleven to thirteen believed their children had not watched online pornography, whereas more than half of their children reported that they had, with almost one in five reporting that they had seen online pornography in the two-week period leading up to the survey (rising to a third of fourteen- to fifteen-year-olds and almost half of sixteen- to seventeen-year-olds). Similar surveys in Australia and the US corroborate these figures.[25]

The UK survey in 2020 found that most children reported feeling upset or disturbed by aggressive or violent pornography they had seen, often accidentally. Girls in particular feared that these types of sexual situations would be normalized among boys and become features of real-life sexual relationships. In the online survey, more than four in ten children agreed that watching it made people "less respectful of the opposite sex."[26]

The Effects of Pornography Use

A plethora of research illustrates the harmful effects of pornography, particularly in terms of its consumption but also to some extent its creation. As awareness of the nature of modern pornography has grown, and as more and more people have become aware of its effects, a number of organizations have sprung up to oppose the industry, to

---

25   For the UK: BBFC, *Young people, Pornography;* Martellozzo et al., "wasn't sure it was normal." For Australia: Lim et al.; Flood and Hamilton, *Youth and Pornography.* For the US: Wright et al., "Exploratory Findings."
26   BBFC.

educate and inform the public, and to support those who have been affected. These include secular and religious organizations from a variety of political and ideological backgrounds, with aims ranging from a complete ban on pornography to the enforcement of some restrictions to explicitly prevent abusive imagery. (I mentioned some of these in the introduction.) Similarly, a number of organizations previously focused on related issues, such as human trafficking, have included pornography as an additional issue on which to campaign or offer support. Many countries have also gained traction on raising awareness of the problem. For example, as I wrote this book in 2021, Germany was seriously considering a national block on at least one major pornography website.

From as early as 1980, the Zillman-Bryant experiments demonstrated how the use of pornography could change attitudes toward sexuality and affect relationships negatively: "Without exception, the more pornography the subjects had viewed . . . the more likely they were to believe others to be sexually active and adventurous . . . [making] gross overestimations of actual sexual practices, according to all available data."[27] Also, pornography, according to one user who participated in the Zillman-Bryant experiments, makes an object out of anybody:

---

27   Paul, *Pornified*, 77–78. Moreover, "60 percent of those who viewed no pornography in the experiment endorsed marriage as 'an important institution'; only 39 percent of those who viewed 'massive' amounts of pornography agreed" (141). And (89) "participants were asked to read a newspaper report about the recent rape of a hitchhiker. . . . Students were then asked to recommend a sentence for the convicted rapist. . . . Men in the 'massive exposure' group recommended an average of 50 months' imprisonment for the rapist, while men who had not viewed the films recommended 95 months" (the figures for the women students were 77 months and 143 months respectively). She also makes the point (91) that what was called "massive exposure" at the time of the study in 1979–80 was already by the time of her book in 2005 not an untypical level of exposure in men who regularly used the internet for pornography, and the material they viewed tended to be significantly more hard-core.

"It takes a three-dimensional human being with feelings—someone who could be your daughter, sister, or mother—and basically says, this is a creature that is only intended to satisfy your sexual desires. It becomes your natural way of thinking. . . . It gets to a point where you can't even look at a woman without first rating her for her physical attributes. You're no longer conscious you're even doing it. It just happens."[28]

We have already mentioned girls' concerns about a negative effect on future sexual relationships with the substantial majority of boys who have significant exposure to pornography. Many documented personal experiences show that a partner's use of pornography contributes to the way they relate sexually, especially, but not only, in terms of the presence of degrading, aggressive, or abusive elements.[29] One such partner said, "Even when he and I were intimate, the sex wasn't intimate. We were two people just sort of taking care of ourselves with each other."[30] Additionally, a rare study that instituted a complete abstinence from pornography use found that just three weeks of abstinence made a positive difference to relationship commitment.[31]

In addition to pornography's effect on relationships, significant evidence also exists of a correlation between pornography use and sexual crime—both quantitative evidence of correlation and anecdotal evidence from serial sexual offenders and murderers.[32] Despite

---

28 Paul, 221. Some researchers describe this phenomenon as a "sexual script" learned from pornography scenes that, as it becomes embedded in the psyche, starts to color real-life experiences. For examples, see Marshall, "Bridging the Theoretical Gap"; Vera-Gray et al., "Sexual violence as a sexual script."

29 See, for example, MacKinnon and Dworkin, *In Harm's Way*; Paul, *Pornified*. Many more reports appear on the websites of the campaigning organizations.

30 Paul, 138.

31 Lambert, "Love That Doesn't Last."

32 For example, Ted Bundy said "the most common interest among serial killers is pornography" (Rieber, *Psychopathology of Language*, 83), and Jeffrey Dahmer, charged with the deaths of seventeen men and boys, told the FBI his

this, the claim of any direct causal link remains controversial, with research continually being published that evidences either side of the argument. Nonetheless, in many jurisdictions, showing a child pornographic material legally constitutes childhood sexual abuse.[33]

In criminal cases, often, the legal standard to demonstrate a link between ill effects and pornography is higher than for other factors. For example, a US court found a company negligently responsible in a sexual assault case for inadequately maintaining the lighting in an underground parking garage. Simple common sense was enough to show that the lack of light was a facilitating factor in the assault, and the court did not need to see "overwhelming scientific research in support of the claim."[34] However, ever since Judge Easterbrook struck down MacKinnon and Dworkin's 1983 antipornography ordinance in Minneapolis, an "overwhelming" degree of scientific evidence is precisely what courts have required in cases where the use of pornography may be alleged as a key contributory factor. This law had been designed to provide legal recourse for women who had suffered specific harm in which pornography was a contributory factor.[35]

One of the particular links between internet pornography and sexual crime that has come into much greater awareness since the 2010s is that among general online pornographic content, there are videos and photographs which have been taken by perpetrators and

---

behavior was motivated by "heavy drinking, pornography, and masturbation" (*Correctional Newsfront*, 7).

33   In the UK, this is part of the definition of sexual abuse according to HM Government (*Working Together to Safeguard Children*, 107). Federal law in the US has been interpreted to include this: "The employment, use, persuasion, inducement, enticement, or coercion of any child to engage in, or assist any other person to engage in, any sexually explicit conduct" (The Child Abuse Prevention and Treatment Act or CAPTA, 42 U.S.C.A. §5106g(a) (4) (202219)). But I am not aware of any court cases that have tested the interpretation.

34   Adams, "Can Pornography Cause Rape?" 13.

35   Mikkola, *Pornography*, 31ff.

observers of sexual abuse. The Internet Watch Foundation was able to confirm 118 illegal instances of child rape and sexual abuse publicly available on one well-known internet pornography site alone between 2017 and 2019,[36] and other cases have been reported in the press.[37] Another type of sexual crime that has come to the attention of the courts involves the use of unwilling participants in the creation of pornography, such as when aspiring models are coerced into taking part in pornographic scenes.[38]

Although the blatant nature of some of these sexual crimes suggests that shame is not such a big issue in sexual matters as it may have been in the past, pornography is nevertheless still associated with shame. Above, I noted that the avoidance of shame is one of the motives of pornography use: it is much easier for me to be shameless if I can be anonymous on the internet and nobody can see what I am doing. Or if I am ashamed of my desires and cannot express them face to face with another person, I may wish to hide my shame in lonely pornography use.

But it turns out that shame does not require another person's judgment—the internal judgment of my own conscience, however buried, is enough. So trying to hide my shame in pornography use

---

36 Many news outlets reported this in 2019–2020, and it also appears on the IWF's website (Puddephatt, "Pornhub").

37 E.g., the BBC reported in 2020 that a teenage victim of a kidnap and rape was extensively recorded on video during the assault, and the footage was uploaded to a pornography site. Complaints to the website yielded no response until the mother of the child posed as a lawyer and threatened legal action (BBC, "'I was raped'").

38 An example widely reported in 2021 was a case where twenty-two young women in the US were coerced and deceived into performing sexual acts on film that were then uploaded to a pornography site (US Dept. of Justice, "Girls-DoPorn Employee"). The young women won a lawsuit, and a federal indictment of the company's owner followed, for the production of child sexual abuse films and trafficking of a minor. At the time of writing, the owner is still wanted on a federal warrant.

can lead to a vicious circle, where shame causes me to turn to pornography, which in turn increases the very shame that led me there in the first place. Shame is its own humiliation, and if I am unable to take positive action to overcome it, and I also suffer from low self-esteem, loneliness, and/or social anxiety, the resulting anger and aggression may manifest in a desire for aggressive or even violent pornography. Even if I do not resort to explicitly aggressive or violent scenes, if I am humiliated and full of shame, pornography will likely be the place where I can with little effort imagine myself in a position of power and dominance.

This has been just a brief survey of some of the aspects of the personal impact of pornography use that have been highlighted in the research. Alongside these, there is additional evidence of effects on psychological and even physical health. For example, one psychological effect some studies have demonstrated is that pornography use reduces the ability to delay gratification (considered a significant predictor of achievement in life).[39] Exercising self-control over pornography use has a stronger effect on strengthening the ability to delay gratification even than exercising control over food (through dieting or fasting). In terms of physical effects, there is anecdotal evidence of recovery from erectile dysfunction after a complete cessation of pornography use for a time.[40]

Despite all the evidence of harm, as I mentioned earlier, there is still some controversy over whether or not there is a causal link between pornography use and sexual crime, or even whether pornography has negative effects on a person's life and relationships. Perhaps a useful comparison is to smoking. Not every smoker gets lung cancer, and some nonsmokers do. This enabled the cigarette industry for

---

39 Negash et al., "Trading Later Rewards."
40 For example, Park et al., "Is Internet Pornography Causing"; Porto, "Habitudes masturbatoires"; Blair, "How difficult is it"; Begovic, "Pornography Induced Erectile Dysfunction."

many years to argue against evidence for a causal link; nevertheless, we widely accept today that there is an established, scientifically validated link—even if the outcome is not the same in all cases.

Not every user of pornography will commit sex crimes or suffer relationship breakdowns. Whether or not this happens depends on a number of factors, of which pornography use is one. What is clear is that pornography use has negative effects in terms of personality, attitudes, relationships, and, of course, spiritual life. Empirical evidence demonstrates this, but it is also implicit within the nature of pornography itself and in the nature of our attraction to it, both as individuals and as a society.

Who Has a Pornography Problem?

Pornography is characterized by lies. It is an imagery of lies, and it leads those who make it, as well as those who view it, to lie. It is an imagery of lies because it portrays, in so many ways, that which is not true. It simulates a relationship where none exists; it presents coerced participants as consenting and willing; it manufactures a simulacrum of pleasure where in fact there is pain, discomfort, and disconnection; it pretends to offer fulfillment and an intimate contact that it cannot provide.

It leads to lies as people justify the profitable business of pornography, which is based on the trauma and abuse of others. It brings forth lies from those who try to justify or hide their use of pornography as well as to hide their internal shame and fear—and this multiplies the lies, since shame and fear are both the cause and the effect of regular pornography use.

Finally, our whole society lies when it pretends pornography has something to do with freedom of action, freedom of relationship, or freedom of speech. And the more I, as a member of this society, continue to accept this state of affairs, the more I also lie to myself if I think I am not implicated in the abuse of others—particularly of the hurt, the weak, the dispossessed, disempowered, and traumatized.

The lies alone show that pornography is a problem for all of us: those who make it, those who use it, those who are in any form of intimate or family relationship with those who use it, those who have children who will marry those who use it, those who have children who will one day be involved in making it, those who have to negotiate its existence and pervasiveness in society—in humor, in comedy, in advertising. In other words, all of us have a pornography problem.

The Zillman-Bryant experiments from 1980 found that people who had been exposed to large amounts of pornography were significantly less likely to want daughters than those who had not. As the journalist Pamela Paul commented, "Who would want their own little girl to be treated that way? Who would want to bring a girl into such a world?"[41] Pornography is a problem for all of us.

Orthodox Christians are no exception: we also cannot escape the problem. When I first began to research this topic back in 2008, I interviewed a number of Orthodox priests who hear confessions. My conversations with clergy and monastics since have confirmed that any Orthodox priest who hears regular confessions will be aware of how common pornography use has become. And neither clergy nor monastics are exempt from temptation themselves.

Pornography is a problem for all of us because *porneia* is the opposite of eros. Therefore, any society that sees nothing wrong with pornography will unlearn the meaning of eros and how to participate in divine eros. Eros is a love that desires an ever fuller and more complete union—as distinct from agape, which is a love that acts for the good of the other. In an icon, eros and agape meet as we cease to be at the center of things and our earthly desires touch

41   Paul, *Pornified*, 80.

another world beyond that immediately visible to our senses. Pornographic images or scenes twist and destroy eros and excise agape. The pornographic image lies about the possibility of eros, as there will never be any real union, and it shows no awareness of agape: here the focus is always on myself, my needs and desires, and the other person exists only as an object for the purpose of meeting those needs and desires.

Separation or Communion

The secular research I outlined above describes how pornography use can change attitudes and habitual ways of relating. This pornographic way of seeing others as objects, as resources for sexual gratification, goes deeper even than that: when we look at another human person as an object, we fail to see them as an icon of Christ, as the image of God. When we deface the image of God in others, we also deface it in ourselves. We cease to meet God in others, and in our failure to meet Christ, our eternal salvation is thrown into question.

In order to move from separation and isolation into relationship and communion, we learn to open ourselves in humility, relate in honesty, and make ourselves vulnerable in front of one another. But in pornography I dominate another; I exercise my own desire and allow the other person no choice, no response, no freedom. I arrogate to myself a power over others I do not have, exchanging the truth of God for a lie. And I cannot console myself even with the belief that the image on my screen is simply unreal. Saint John of Damascus reminds us that to insult the image is to insult the prototype[42] (that is, the person the image portrays), just as in an icon, to venerate the

---

42   John of Damascus, *Three Treatises*, Treatise II.61, 78–79: "If you insult the image of the emperor, you carry your insult to the archetype of this dignity . . . the insult borne to the emperor's image entails insult to the emperor himself."

image is to venerate the prototype. The prototype of the image that is every human being is God.[43]

An icon is holy because it connects us to the reality of the image it portrays. Pornography, in contrast, reifies our separation from the real person represented in the image. Father John Breck describes pornography as "demonic iconography," saying that instead of feeding the mind and soul with heavenly food as iconography does, it "infests the mind with corrupt images that produce corruption in the depths of the soul."[44] And it is not enough to empty ourselves of corrupt images and vain visions, separating ourselves from them; we need also to fill our minds with healthy images and with icons of truth that nourish our minds and souls, uniting our souls with what is good, true, and beautiful. Otherwise, clearing out one demon will leave our soul open for many more (Matt. 12:43–45).

The icon exists to draw us into deeper communion; the image is a window that we can pass through to a deeper reality. Pornography exists as a substitute for communion, as a supposed easy way to gain the pleasure without the struggle of relating to another human being. In pornography there is nothing to pass through and no deeper reality to find—quite the opposite. Pornography strips a human person, an icon of Christ, of that iconographic nature, as the spirit is separated from the flesh and the flesh presented as a commodity, as an end in itself. Do any of us wish to live in a society where this is the accepted norm and is seen as the ultimate reality?

In fact, while the icon brings me to a person, pornography begins to damage my very ability to relate on a personal level, since in pornography human beings are often interchangeable so long as they match a particular type. If I use pornography, I exchange the person for a stereotype, meaning that I fail to see not only the personhood

---

43   John of Damascus, Treatise III.73, 125.

44   Breck, *Sacred Gift of Life*, 103.

of the one portrayed but also my own. Thus I destroy any possibility of interrelationship. When we come to venerate an icon, on the other hand, although we are not looking at a physically literal image (as in a simple photographic image), we are being invited to see with the eyes of love. We are provided with the freedom of a personal encounter that transcends physical necessity, as we see the portrayed other (the saint in the icon) in all his or her unique and eternal beauty.[45] Using pornography, in fact, is a direct manifestation of Davor Dzalto's characterization of the Fall, where "human beings become what they choose to be—things and facts of an objectivized and naturalized world, with no unmediated part in the life of God, except through the icon."[46]

So the way we begin to purify our vision and our desires is by venerating the holy icons, venerating with our whole selves—body, mind, and spirit. Sometimes I may feel unworthy to approach the saint in the icon because of the impurity of my soul, but this is backwards: I need to start with veneration, and that is the path to finding purity.

Saint John of Damascus[47] wrote about a demon of lust who promised to leave a great recluse in peace if he would only stop venerating the icon of the Theotokos. When he confessed this to an elder, the elder told him, "It would be better for you to leave no brothel in this town unentered than to refuse to venerate our Lord and God Jesus Christ together with His own Mother." The primary purpose of the demon of lust was not to tempt the monk to sexual immorality—though this was part of the process—but to prevent the monk from venerating the icon. Learning from this, I find that my primary

---

45   This insight comes from Boss, *Empress and Handmaid*, 5–6. There's also something here about personal freedom and the possibility of a relationship of love and veneration transcending the necessity of the fallen physical world.

46   Dzalto, *Human Work of Art*, 56.

47   John of Damascus, *Three Treatises,* Treatise, 1.64, 55–56, citing a story from John Moschus's *Spiritual Meadow.*

purpose is not to attempt to rid myself of pornography or the porni-fied worldview, but to lay that aside (as in the Liturgy we lay aside all earthly cares). It is when we learn how to truly venerate the holy icons that we can participate in the holiness they offer and gain the true gift of sight.

PART 2

Masks

Have you hardened your hearts? Having eyes, do you not see?
—Mark 8:17–18

CHAPTER 3

Becoming Aware of Masks

I SAID IN THE PREVIOUS chapter that learning to live in communion requires me to open myself to the other. When I talk about
masks, I am speaking of the way in which I find myself unable to do
this, unable to see and be seen in truth. My mask refers to the physical and psychological aspects of my way of being that hide my deeper
emotional and spiritual self, and keep others hidden from me. I may
have a collection of masks, each of which has its appealing shiny outer
layers and its shadowy underlayers.

Most visible to others is the shiny surface of the mask I wear,
which I construct (either consciously or unconsciously) by painting
on it the face I would like to have: the face I would like others to see
and know me by. This makes it harder for others to perceive me as I
truly am—to see me iconographically. But underneath this shiny and
brightly painted outer mask, there are darker layers—shadowy layers
on which my characteristic sins and temptations are painted.

Every mask covers the true image of God in me. Because of the
masks with all their layers of paint, I cannot be seen as I truly am,
and even I myself cannot see His true likeness in me. And as we are
relational beings by nature, the ability or inability to see and be seen
works from both sides. This means that when I look at another person,

or at any part of God's creation, because of the spiritual blindness the layers of my masks have created, I fail to see and therefore cannot truly encounter the other. In fact, even if the other's true image is barely covered by the thinnest and most translucent of veils, because of my blindness it will be as if they too are behind the thickest and most opaque of masks. Trapped behind my masks, I see others, to a greater or lesser degree, not as people in their own right but as projections arising from the reflection of myself in the masks' shiny surface.

On the other hand, when another looks at me, those with more perceptive eyes will see through even the shiniest and most brightly painted surface layer of my mask and discern some of the dark, shadowy paintings of my sins beneath. To the most perceptive eyes, my mask as a whole will be as thin as gossamer; those eyes will still be able to see me behind all the layers. And this is the challenge of the Christian life: to learn instinctively to walk according to the spirit, in order to see the deeper reality behind the masks or beyond the flesh.

Saint Paul mentions this in his letter to the Romans when he talks about perceiving the invisible spiritual world through the physical world: "There is no condemnation for those in Christ Jesus who do not walk according to the flesh but according to the spirit. . . . For the *phronema* of the flesh is death but the phronema of the spirit is life and peace" (Rom. 8:1, 6). The word *phronema*, usually translated into English as *mind*, means the mind-spirit-ethos rather than the intellectual or cognitive mind. This is important because we may instinctively believe here that we have to keep *thinking* about the Spirit. However, St. Paul is saying that we need to orient our *whole being* toward the Spirit—to develop a habit of uniting our body, mind, and spirit to instinctively see, experience, and understand the physical world in the fuller context of the spiritual.

What Saint Paul refers to here as the *flesh* is what I am referring to as masks. *Mask* in this sense is the flesh when it is cut off from the life-giving spirit—when it is the "body of death," as St. Paul also calls it:

> I do not know what I am accomplishing! . . . I do not do the good I want, but the bad I do not want is what I do in practice! . . . What a wretched person I am! Who will deliver me from this body of death? I thank God through our Lord Jesus Christ! (Rom. 7:15, 19, 24–25)

Saint Paul here associates the mask—the body of death—with repeatedly doing the evil I want to avoid doing. This is probably a recognizable experience to many of us, as we return again and again to confess the same sins. It is also a pretty good description of addiction. I so much want something better; I decide with determination to change, not to indulge the addiction again, but then somehow, despite this desire and resolution, I still give in to the temptation. Habitual behavior is hard to change, and it is easy to get disheartened. And then the feeling of failure makes me even more vulnerable to giving in to temptation, as the demons whisper into my mind that giving in will make it all feel better . . . and it doesn't matter if I do it just one more time.

I keep coming back to these habits because I have a real need. But my real need is hidden behind my masks: I can't access it fully, and I do not know what will really fulfill it, so I keep coming back to the substitutes, the misdirection of the masks. These lesser desires— these shadowy images painted under the bright, shiny surface— are related to the real need. They are a symbol of the real need, but because they are substitutes, they can never fulfill me. My resolutions to change my habits cannot work, because I cannot wish the need away. Willingness to change, in itself, is not enough. Without both the willingness and the ability to see beyond the mask, I will be stuck in the addictive loop. The best I can do is resolve to do something that will "improve" me superficially—but this may do nothing more than polish and beautify my mask.

My desires are so conflicted. Even when I know Christ, I am still tempted to listen to the whispered words of those demons rather than the true Word, which is Christ. I am still tempted to give in to the dead-end desires that underlie the polished and brightly painted masks, which miss the mark of truth and ultimately push me away from Christ and the fullness of all truth and life. Indulging these lesser desires directly is counterproductive, however—not only because it can't fulfill the deeper need but also because the pleasure it does give forms a greater temptation to return to it. In this sense, it continually reinforces a loss of hope, a form of despair: now I am going to return to this pleasure because it seems the desire can never truly be fulfilled, and this mask is the best I am going to get, even though it is a counterfeit of that deeper fulfillment.

This pattern is particularly obvious in pornography, so why might I want to use pornography even if I already know this? I use it because I want things I can't easily get another way (all those things I discussed in previous chapters as the reasons people use pornography), or I use it to avoid the dangers of a true and deep relationship, which, para-doxically, is what I really desire. The mask is a caricature of the face I really desire but in my despair cannot hope to access. But accepting the mask and becoming comfortable with it makes me less and less able or willing to seek out or even remember the existence of the pure face my deepest soul cries out for.

There are many examples that demonstrate how expressing my desire ends up driving away the possibility of its fulfillment. For example, we have probably all seen or experienced a one-sided rela-tionship in which one person pursues another. If I am the pursuer, my desire becomes increasingly desperate until it becomes the kind of neediness that repulses the person I desire and wish to attract. Instead of offering myself as a gift, I force myself on the other person, and in the end this precludes the possibility of knowing and being known. There is nothing wrong with the basic desire, the longing, but the more I try to follow that desire, the more I destroy the possibility of its fulfillment. This loss only serves to deepen the need, and so the pattern of relating can become a vicious circle, a destructive habitual way of relating. People who know and love me may say to me, "But this isn't really you." They perceive that they are seeing a mask instead of my true face. I also lose the true face of the other in the obsession and in the other's reaction to the obsession.

So again, whether or not I have an addiction to pornography in the usual understanding of the expression, I realize that I have my own parallel temptations and misdirected desires. And if I fail to see the world iconographically, there is a sense in which I am habitually seeing it pornographically, because I am not seeing what is behind the masks, or maybe I am not even aware that the masks I see are not all there is. Healing begins with becoming aware of my own masks, my "body of death"—both the masks I create for myself and those I impose on others.

My masks present a picture that is unfaithful to my true reality—in this sense they are *porno-graphic*. However, like all pornographic imagery, my masks do have meaning and can be understood. There is nothing that *is* that does not have meaning, since in order to exist at all, my masks must maintain some connection to the Source of All Life, who is also the Source of All Truth. If I learn to be aware of my masks, to see what is painted on them, I will begin to see that the designs on them (shiny and shadowy layers) actually symbolize my deeper and more intimate needs and desires.

In this section, in the chapters that follow, we will consider more closely three of these shadowy layers of my masks that are particularly relevant to pornography: lust, shame, and fantasy. These illustrate some of the characteristics of masks I have already alluded to—that they are flesh disconnected from the spirit of life, delusions that drive us from all truth, and ultimately a mockery of God, deny-ing our dependence on Him. Examining what these layers look like can help us become aware of our own masks. As we become aware of them, we can begin to learn how to see past them by living out in our own lives a pattern of venerating rather than objectifying, and a pattern of overcoming addiction (the repeated seeking of pleasure or of feeling good), so that we can desire *truly*, which means to seek after true and deep joy. In other words, we can help ourselves or others only if we learn first to be aware of the masks and then to see beyond or through them.

A Prayer for True and Deep Joy

Blessed are You, O Lord, teach me Your statutes.
I am the image of Your ineffable glory
Though I bear the marks of straying:
Have compassion for Your creature, O Master
And purify me by Your loving-kindness;
Grant me the homeland of my heart's desire,
Making me again a citizen of Paradise.[1]

---

1   From the Evlogitaria of the Departed, my translation.

CHAPTER 4

Lust: The Decaying Body of Love without Its Soul

L UST IS NOTHING OTHER THAN shadowy images on a mask, but it tempts me to see the world pornographically. Becoming aware of lust is central to understanding why I get caught up in habits I find difficult to break. Lust is the decaying body of love without its soul. Lust is where I end up when the physical has been isolated from deeper spiritual reality; it is made up only of images on masks that misdirect and obscure the possibility of love, which is hidden away behind. Lust is the passion that arises when a desire that *in truth* would direct me to a real relationship of mutual love has been misdirected and truncated *in fact* so that sating the desire can never ultimately fulfill me.

At the same time, lust is about habit and addiction—I like the "feel good," the pleasure, and I want more of it because it masks my pain and my fears. The fruit that invites me to pluck it is so enticing, promising to fulfill what it can't. And even though I know this, I still feel the blood rushing to my head when I even think about indulging my temptation. Ultimately, I hide behind masks of lust because I am afraid to love. I am afraid to be vulnerable, afraid of getting hurt, of getting lost; I am afraid of getting tied down in commitment and responsibility. Vulnerability, by definition, is risky and takes courage, but I need to address this fear in order to have any hope of coming out from behind my masks.

Again, the question is about transforming and reorienting my desires. I am able to find purity in transformation, not in closing my desires down. Not in suppressing my passions, but in transcending them. The aim is not to become stoic but to live fully. And I don't want to clean out the house of my soul only to provide it as a house for some new demons (Matt. 12:43–45); I want to fill it with holy desire so that I can be united with the ultimate source of true joy.

Purity is about putting on a wedding garment and going to a feast, a party (Matt. 22:1–14). Purity is about freedom from prison, not locking myself or my desires down. That which is locked down inside will almost certainly come out eventually, and it is what comes out of me that makes me impure, as Christ says:

> "That which goes forth out of the person is what defiles the person. For from within, out of people's hearts, ugly thoughts [dialogismoi] go forth: adulteries, sexual unfaithfulnesses [porneiai], murders, thefts, greeds, iniquities, deceit, lechery, evil eye, blasphemy, arrogance, mindlessness. All these evil things from within go forth and defile the person." (Mark 7:20–23)

And if these evil things do not emerge and go forth directly, they continue to distort the person from within—which in turn affects how that person sees the world and all relationships. This is therefore still a case of the evil things going forth, but in a less direct way.

That evil eye comes from within the heart—the eye that sees pornographically, the eye of lust for sex, of lust for wealth and/or power.

But the eye of our hearts is really designed to see iconologically. This, the true eye of the heart, is called the *nous* in Greek. The nous (which, rather confusingly, is, like the word *phronema* in the previous chapter, also commonly translated into English as *mind*) is that power of the heart or soul that connects us to God, and purity is the context that enables us to see with that true eye, as we see in Matthew 5:8: "Blessed are the pure in heart, for they shall see God." Later in the Sermon on the Mount, the Lord also says, "If your eye is pure then your whole body will be shining; but if your eye is evil then your whole body will be dark" (Matt. 6:22–23).

The Church Fathers also talk about the purification of the eye. Saint Gregory of Nyssa says that the person who purifies the eye of the soul will perceive the image of God within.[1] To this end, St. Augustine says:

> Our whole business then, Brethren, in this life is to heal this eye of the heart whereby God may be seen. To this end are celebrated the Holy Mysteries; to this end is preached the word of God; to this end are the moral exhortations of the Church, those, that is, that relate to the correction of manners, to the amendment of carnal lusts, to the renouncing [of] the world, not in word only, but in a change of life: to this end is directed the whole aim of the Divine and Holy Scriptures, that that inner man may be purged of that which hinders us from the sight of God.[2]

Or as St. Isaac the Syrian neatly sums it up: "This life has been given to you for repentance; do not waste it in vain pursuits."[3] The ascetic path aims at quieting and guarding the heart so that these *logismoi*,

---

1   Gregory of Nyssa, *Lord's Prayer*, 148.
2   Sermon 38 on the New Testament, para. 5. Schaff, NPNF-I, 6:380.
3   Isaac the Syrian, *Ascetical Homilies*, 364.

these evil thoughts, do not arise. And according to Metropolitan Hierotheos, "When the Fathers speak of 'thoughts' (logismoi), they do not mean simple thoughts, but the images and representations behind which there are always appropriate thoughts."[4] He goes on to explain that logismoi form within us when simple images of things or people are joined with passions in our heart.

We learn, then, that these things are inseparable: repentance, purity, and a clear eye of the heart—the nous that connects us to God and enables us to see truly, to perceive the unseen, to see through the veils, to take off the masks of lust and indeed the masks of all the passions. This is a big turnabout, a significant reorientation, which is what the word *repentance* means, of course.

And this is what iconography is about: a reorientation from lust to pure love, from the misleading logismoi (evil thoughts) to the true *logoi* (words that are true icons of the Logos, the Word that is Christ). This reorientation is a vital part of an iconological approach to the world, which is necessarily other-centric. The vanishing point of the icon's perspective throws me into relief against the primary focus on the other: I learn to see myself as I am reflected through others and the other[5] (other people, all of creation, and ultimately God) rather than looking at others and seeing a reflection or projection of myself. In contrast, the iconoclastic and idolatrous viewpoints—those that cannot see beyond the mask—are egocentric. From the viewpoint of my lust mask, I appear to be more than I really am, but the other

---

4   Hierotheos, *Orthodox Psychotherapy*, 215.
5   It is important to note here that this requires wisdom and discretion—I do not necessarily see the truth of me reflected back in fallen creation: sometimes the image of me reflected back will be distorted. The opposite danger here is to lose myself in others and in their own distorted images of me. But even when a distorted image of me is reflected back, there is still something to learn, because (by definition) behind every distorted image is a true image. Wisdom comes in being able to see what that veiled or masked true image reveals of me.

appears to be only what he, she, or it is *in fact*. In other words, I do not allow others to transcend their physical bodies; I do not recognize them as images of God to venerate, while at the same time seeing myself as much more than my physical body alone and not being aware of the way in which my objectifying anti-communion way of being is actually reducing my personhood.

Iconoclasm and idolatry are different in that iconoclasm seeks purity by destroying the possibility of rousing the passions through imagery, whereas idolatry focuses on connecting with the physical world, imagining it to possess in itself the power and meaning that in truth are only reflected from its Creator. Nevertheless, iconoclasm and idolatry share a horror of the Incarnation, not only as a reality but even as a concept. Any non-iconological worldview either sees the physical world as unable to participate in the divine (because even the idea that the divine could interpenetrate the physical is disgusting), or it worships the physical world for its own sake (because the idea that there needs to be something greater beyond what I sense is not only ridiculous but dangerous and possibly insane). In either case, the key commonality is the absence of the union of Word and flesh.

But it is precisely this union of Word and flesh that is necessary to transcend lust and transform it into love. It may be that both iconoclast and idolater are reacting to the same lust masks in different ways. The iconoclast may be terrified of the power of the lust masks and is therefore afraid of the flesh, hates it, or has contempt for it, whereas the idolater lusts after it, worships it, or hopes for fulfillment through it. The arguments about pornography frequently occur between the former and the latter groups—the puritans and the hedonists (who may prefer to self-describe as the "decent" and the "sex-positive," respectively). Yet to the pure, all things are pure. If we had a truly iconological soul, we would not be defiled, and lust would have no hold over us.

It may be that it is more difficult to escape addictive patterns of lust as modern media and technological imagery have intensified the manipulation of reality and the image's ability to break the iconological link with reality. In that sense, as Jean-Luc Marion says, we see "our world in its accomplished state of idolatry."[6] At this level of disconnect from reality, there is little to challenge the fantasy. In fact, it may be that lusting after internet pornography and its associated fantasies is actually even worse than physical sexual sin with another person. Jesus says it is at least as bad to look with lust as to commit adultery (Matt. 5:27–28). But even if it is lust that leads me to meet another person in their physical reality, when I connect with them physically, I cannot avoid encountering them at least to some degree in all their reality. Since we are both real people, each made up of an inseparable body, mind, and spirit, if I develop a physical relationship with that other person, it must contain at least some elements of a mind and spirit relationship too.

And if such a connection lasts beyond a single sexual act, the reality behind the lust mask intensifies, and it is possible for it to then take on some of the aspects of love—through the relationship, I begin to learn to see what lies behind the masks. This is all impossible with image-based (mask-based) lust, wherein the object of lust is and always remains to me a fantasy, entirely detached from reality, and I never encounter a real person. It is more dangerous to embark on the real-life physical relationship because of the vulnerability and risk involved, as we saw earlier in this chapter. But the physical relationship at least has the potential to become more salvific, since it enables some kind of taste of real union.

Nevertheless, even a real-life interpersonal and physical relationship does not guarantee an escape from the mask, as is clear in the story of Samson and Delilah. Samson's lust for Delilah meant

---

6   Marion, *Crossing*, 82.

that instead of seeing the reality of her motives, he saw only the mask of his own pleasure. From this blindness, he lost the source of divine strength God had blessed him with. Moreover, his spiritual and relational blindness became also a physical blindness when the Philistines violently gouged out his eyes (Judg. 16:21). Ironically, it is Delilah's betrayal that leads to his physical blindness but also enables him to begin to see how he has been taken in by the mask of lust.

How might Samson have told his story, while he was in that relationship with Delilah? And what stories might I tell when I am involved in my pornographic lies? Just like Samson's story, my stories are the stories of my masks, not of my deeper self. Similarly, all who make pornography or have made it in the past have their own stories, the stories of their own masks. And then, how might Delilah have talked about her relationship with Samson? Would she have claimed to love him? Or would she have laughed at him behind his back? Or both? Which version of the story might she have believed? And how might Samson have told his story once he was faced with the finished fact of Delilah's betrayal? This would probably have been quite a different story from the one he would have told earlier.

We all tell our own stories, at least to ourselves if not to others, and we draw on these stories for our interpretations of our lives and relationships, and to make sense of the world around us. Our stories in this sense all have morals. It is through telling our stories that we make our sorrows bearable, and this storytelling is necessary. But even if I cannot tell the true story in words and tell only the stories of my masks, my life will write the true stories iconographically anyway, to those who have eyes to see. All masks, like all icons, tell stories—they are written as much as drawn or painted. If I am drawn to pornography, this can be understood iconologically as a telling of my story: it tells perhaps of how I cannot connect to my life's deeper purpose, and how I lack connection and fulfillment as a result. Or it tells of past experiences of sexual, physical, or emotional abuse. Or it tells of broken relationships and a life bearing an enormous weight of disconnection, loneliness, or shame.

Similarly, the way I look at the world tells the story of how the world has related to me. At the opening of the introduction to this book, I quoted the words of a former porn actor who said that pornography is a soul-destroying industry and that he went into it because he wanted his soul destroyed. In the course of the conversations recorded in the chat, he also talked about some of the trauma of his early life. Many of those involved in making pornography have experienced abuse and trauma in their lives before they got into pornography. In this way, the porn tells their story—a story of abuse, trauma, and powerlessness. A story of darkness and destruction, and of the way we may go on to be drawn into the darkness and destruction repeatedly.

Even though this telling of the story is factual, it is nevertheless still a mask, covering a yet deeper truth. The abuse, trauma, darkness, and destruction, the lies, heartbreak, and violence are not for any of us a true story of who we are as people. They are *facts* about our lives; they have affected everything about who we are and how we relate to others—but they are not ultimate *truths*. Either consciously or unconsciously, we hide and protect under our masks the truth of who we are as people because life has proved too dangerous for us ever to consider showing our real selves. Every time we have started to show our real selves, we have suffered for it, and it is an entirely rational reaction therefore to hide. And yet if we stay behind the mask of lust, we can never be truly seen for who we are, and we can never make those real connections that we desire.

In order to make those real connections, we need to be able to tell the stories of our heart. Saint Macarius gives us a vivid picture of the heart, where we store up all our life's experience:

The heart itself is but a little vessel, and yet there are dragons, and there lions, and there venomous beasts, and all the treasures of wickedness; and there are rough uneven ways, there chasms; there likewise is God, there the angels, there life and the kingdom, there light and the apostles, there the heavenly cities, there the treasures, there are all things.[7]

I may be consciously aware of some of what is in my heart, but much of it I am not aware of. I do not want to go down amidst the dragons and the poisonous beasts that lurk within, and so I may want to mask those things and reinterpret my story in a way that is more comforting—a way I can live with.

In this way, the story I tell will become a form of objectification, because I am desperate to fix in place something that will make sense for me, something that will preclude unknowing and that will enable me in my powerlessness to gain power over the world by controlling at least my own understanding of it. In a similar way, when I look at others, instead of relating to them in truth and mutual vulnerability, I see a mask that the eye of my heart draws over their true faces. A vivid representation of this type of objectification is the painting *The Rape* by René Magritte, where what appears to be the face of a woman is actually a representation of her naked torso (please note: this is a highly disturbing image).

As I become accustomed to objectifying, the more I expose myself to pornography, the more I see the rest of the world as pornographic. This is the opposite of the process of purification, where the eye of my heart learns to see what lies beyond the flesh. In this increasingly pornified view, I see the flesh everywhere, and I increasingly objectify the people I encounter. Objectified by my

---

7   Mason, *Fifty Spiritual Homilies*, Homily XLIII.7, 272–273.

mask of lust, the sexual element is more present, an ever-greater fea-
ture in my awareness of others. My interpretations of words, tones
of voice, glances, and movements are all affected. This is a spiritual
process of increasing blindness, and the neurological process of
neuroplasticity[8] reflects this spiritual reality physically: the pathways and connections that I exercise in my brain get stronger, and
the ones I do not use become weaker.

This process expands across my life. What I have put into my mind
and my soul will form the drawings on both my own masks and the
masks I impose on others. It will be the content of my stories and the
way I interpret the world. It will influence the way I interpret texts,
stories, and history. It will dictate what I infer from all kinds of hints,
and it will mean that suggestion will become suggestive. It will even
affect silence. Silence can be full (and Foucault rightly points out[9]
that we can use silence to communicate as effectively as words, if not
more so). But silence can also be empty. Either way, it does not preclude me from projecting my own meanings onto it. In this way, the
mask I impose on others becomes also a mirror, as what is inside me
becomes the way I interpret the person I see. If only I had the eyes to
see that it is in fact the darkness in myself that I see shadowing the
other's face.

These masks, then, are the result of sin: my sin, the sins of others,
and the fallen nature of the world. I sometimes think I can have a little individual sin I keep to myself, but this is impossible, as each sin
changes the image not only on the mask I show to others but also on
the masks I see over their faces. In fact, every little sin I hide in secret
is of cosmic significance, as St. Sophrony says:

---

8   The ability of the brain to change. This will be discussed further in chapter 8.
    See also Doidge, *Brain That Changes*.

9   Foucault, in *History of Sexuality* Vol. 1. The theme of the use of silence runs
    throughout the book.

The essence of sin consists not in the infringement of ethical standards but in a falling away from the eternal Divine life for which man was created and to which, by his very nature, he is called. . . . The sin of our forefather Adam was not the only sin of cosmic significance. Every sin, manifest or secret, committed by each one of us affects the rest of the universe.

He goes on to explain this further:

Sin is committed first of all in the secret depths of the human spirit but its consequences involve the individual as a whole. A sin will reflect on a man's psychological and physical condition, on his outward appearance, on his personal destiny. Sin will, inevitably, pass beyond the boundaries of the sinner's individual life, to burden all humanity and thus affect the fate of the whole world.[10]

Thus, sin affects everything. It affects what I see and what others see in me. The mask of sin prevents me from seeing clearly, and whatever my intellectual beliefs may be, it makes me functionally an iconoclast. And pornography, ultimately, is an inevitable result of iconoclasm. If I disconnect myself from the world around me, I cannot see iconologically. If I cannot perceive the truth behind the veil (if I cannot even simply know that there is a behind-the-veil; if I am not aware that creation *is* a veil), then my only alternative is to believe that what is materially before me is its own meaning—that it is all there is. Thus, I cannot really see love but only lust. As a human being I may still intuit the existence of love, but if I cannot perceive anything beyond the veil, I may come to believe that love and faithfulness are not truly real, that they are just metaphorical or imaginary

---

10   Sophrony, *Saint Silouan*, 31.

constructs that we use as a sort of "legal fiction" to regulate sex, which is itself what we must really be looking for. That is a materialist, pornological way of seeing.

The iconological way of seeing is radically different. As *iconophiles*—or more accurately *iconodules*—we know that what we see is only a small part of what really is: just the tip of the iceberg. Once we learn to see iconologically, masks no longer fool us, and as we begin to perceive the masks, and then to perceive what lies behind the masks, they start to become more like veils. What lies behind the veil remains veiled from us because we are not yet strong enough to see—like Moses, who had to hide in the cleft of the rock as God passed, because no one can see the face of God and live (Ex. 33:20–23).

But seeing iconologically allows us to begin to perceive the face of God through the veils even while we know we are unable to fully face the Reality. Seeing iconologically implies the humility of knowing how far we are from being ready to see that Reality directly, face to face. As St. Paul puts it in 1 Corinthians 13:12: "We see now through a mirror, obscurely." Seeing iconologically implies that repentance (not vain pursuits) should be our way of life. Through repentance we can purify the lustful eyes of our hearts so that we gain the ability to see more fully. Seeing iconologically implies that we understand the significance of our lives, as everything we say, think, or do affects a reality much greater and deeper than we can know. Seeing iconologically implies that neither our genetic inheritance nor our physical environment ultimately determines who we are and what we do—that although these affect us, we have a freedom that goes far, far deeper than we can imagine.

A Prayer of St. Paul[11]

I pray
that the God of our Lord Jesus Christ, the Father of glory,
give you a spirit of wisdom and revelation
in the full knowledge of Him.
Having the eyes of your heart enlightened,
may you come to know the hope of His calling
and the wealth of the glory of His inheritance in the saints.

---

11 Ephesians 1:17–18 follows "I pray."

CHAPTER 5

Shame: The Delusion That Death Is Victorious

S HAME, LIKE LUST, IS PAINTED on the shadowy layers of my masks beneath the shiny surface—thus, I may not be fully aware of shame even when I feel it. I may experience it as feeling unlovable, inadequate, or worthless. I may experience it as that lonely feeling that I should not share something of myself, since it seems that others will only meet it with judgment and never with understanding. Or I may experience it as a memory of an embarrassing situation long in the past that still gives me nightmares because this embarrassment somehow strikes at the root of who I think I am.

Shame has many possible sources. My shame may be related to past abuse. It may be associated with my perception that I am unable to live up to my potential. It may be related to my perceived failure in relationships, in work, or in any part of life. It may be related to any great disappointment or loss in my life. But whatever it is related to, it inevitably leads me to cover it with a mask. I fit the mask to cover my shame: to protect me from others, but also to protect me from myself.

With my masks of shame, even when I go to confession, I don't really know how to confess, and I only let out some small pieces of carefully controlled information about my experience. Everything else I keep hidden behind the masks. All the hurts, the resentments,

66

the anger, the tears—I cram all this into the tiny and ever-shrinking space behind the masks. Desires I have that I know I shouldn't try to meet externally, with other people, I keep behind my masks. Memories of the times I have acted out. Fantasies of acting out desires that I dare not try to fulfill in practice. Things I feel I can't search out in words, images, or actions—I keep them all behind the masks.

All this shame means I cannot risk having the masks slip because I could not endure the self-exposure that would entail; so my masks of shame become a source of much anxiety. I expend a great deal of subconscious energy making sure the masks firmly cover my truer face. In the depths of my shame, I am stuck because I am desperate to be seen but also desperate to hold the protective masks in place—and these are incompatible desires. I am anxious, I am exhausted, I am in despair, and all hope is gone. All I can do is keep on going, holding the masks. I exist, but I am not able to live. In such a state, I make my heartfelt cry with the psalmist:

O Lord God of my salvation,
By day I have cried and by night, facing You.
Accept my prayer before You,
Bend Your ear to my petition.
Because my soul is filled with ugliness,
And my life draws near to Hades.
I am counted with those going down into the pit,
I am become as a person helpless, free among the dead.
Like the slain sleeping in the grave,
The ones You do not still remember
Who are rejected out of Your hand.
(Ps. 87:2–6)[1]

---

1   Ps. 88:1–5 in translations from the Hebrew text.

Behind the masks of shame, my true self is indeed cut off and lies helpless in the hell of my own shame and disconnectedness. I feel that nothing can get better, that it is not worth fighting anymore, that there is no possibility of real, deep relationship. I am convinced the idea that the beginning of some ultimate, heavenly union is possible in this awful earthly life is an impossible dream. How can I exist in this hell and not despair? But despair at its most all-consuming is incompatible with life. And yet, what hell awaits me if I die?

The depth of this experience of desolation in shame is sometimes contrasted with guilt.[2] In this understanding, *guilt* refers to my awareness that I have committed some kind of sin in thought, word, or deed. I feel uncomfortable about this incongruence with what I believe and with the person I would like to be, and that enables me to reflect, repent where necessary, and live on. *Shame,* on the other hand, occurs when I cannot distinguish my sin in thought, word, or deed from my true nature: in shame it seems to me (consciously or unconsciously) that the sin reflects who I really am in the depths of my heart. In this sense, it points to the shattered condition of the image of God in me, and it can mean that I see myself as utterly cut off from God and from all goodness: forsaken among the dead, helpless, like the slain that lie in the grave, like those whom God remembers no more.

In practice, the words *shame* and *guilt* are often used interchangeably. Alternatively, people sometimes make a similar distinction to the one I have described above by contrasting the concept of *healthy shame* with *toxic shame*. But whichever word or expression we use, there is a distinction in meaning that is important: the difference between, on the one hand, my awareness of my *sin*—of times when I have *missed the mark* of reflecting God's likeness—and on the other

---

2   For example, Brené Brown in *Daring Greatly* draws a contrast between guilt over a specific issue that I see as distinct from my personhood, versus shame which defines who I am.

hand, the feeling that I am entirely cut off from God and rotten to the core.

Once we have learned to understand creation iconologically, we know that while we live, we always continue to bear the image of God. In the depths of our hearts, this is always who we really are. While we continue to draw breath, the ultimate reality we all reflect is God's life, and that is a life of perfect goodness and love. Deep down beyond the dragons and all the other "treasures of wickedness"[3] in the heart, it is the image of God that most truly defines who we are. However obscured that image may seem, it is possible to read my particular shame iconologically to help find my way through my heart—past the dragons and back to Him.

So if I have experienced, for example, the passion of anger inside, and if I have gone on to express it, usually I feel guilt (or a healthy kind of shame) for having betrayed my vocation of living a Christlike life, and I can turn to God in repentance. I will confess, be forgiven, receive forgiveness, and try again. But sometimes I experience some temptation—such as a sexual temptation—and I express it or act on it, or even just think about it, and this time, somehow the shame I feel is not healthy. It is toxic—that is, it can overwhelm my ability to deal with it, to find healing. It can overwhelm me as a person. In such a case, instead of feeling that I have betrayed my vocation and that I can repent, I somehow feel as though my vocation is completely destroyed—as though the possibility of ever being able to turn back to Christ is destroyed. And even if I have not acted out, the ongoing desires or fears—just the temptations alone—can give me this impression. And if what happened to me was not my fault—for example, if I was a victim of sexual abuse—even then I may feel that same toxic shame that seems to close off the avenue back to God and lock me behind my masks.

---

3   Mason, *Fifty Spiritual Homilies*, Homily XLIII.7, 272–273.

In shame I feel that the sin is part of me—I am unable to separate myself from it. Many sins do not have this effect on me, though in any sin, there is an element of union with the demonic. My mind spots the little thought, the temptation, hovering around, and rather than saying "Get thee behind Me, Satan" (Matt. 16:23, KJV), I allow the thought to entertain or entrance me, and I let it land in my mind. By entertaining it there, I give it a home in me, and as it becomes at home in my mind, it also becomes at home in my body through my actions. However, with many sins, afterward I am still able to see the sin as separate from me, whereas in shame I cannot make this distinction with my whole being, even if I understand it theoretically in my mind. If I am not suffering from this toxic kind of shame, I can see my sin as a result of a temptation to do something essentially foreign to my nature as a person whom God has created in His image. I can disown the sin, let it go, and hope that next time I will learn the strength not to be attracted to the sin from the first moment.

However, sometimes, and especially with sexual sins, I am not able to let the sin go in this way—and this is the domain of shame. Sexuality is an icon of union and communion, and on some level we feel this deeply. We experience an inappropriate sexual act or encounter as a union outside God or apart from God—a union that is a direct challenge to our union and communion with God, an unfaithful union, a *pornographic* union. And it is a union that I have enacted not only in my soul but also in my body: as a whole person, I have turned away from God, or been turned away from God, because of this union, which is in some way apart from His love.

So then, in opposition to the true nature of sexuality, it is a lonely experience, this sexual sin, this inappropriate sexual experience—even if it is a case of sexual abuse and I am the innocent, abused one rather than the perpetrator. These experiences of sexuality have one way or another incorporated a demonic element into the natural God-given expression of sexuality as an icon of union and communion in Him. Because this sexual experience unites me with someone or something apart from God and seems to cut me off from God, it leaves me to some degree alone. It seems I have no one to turn to. I have so much shame, I feel as if I cannot even turn to God; either my desire or my experience or both seem to have made even this impossible.

And yet, this feeling too is iconological: in reality, the very feeling of shame as separation is in itself an experience of God's love. God's love for me is not moving away or diminishing; rather, I feel myself being seduced, led, or dragged away from that source of light and communion in Him. I feel unable to turn back to the love that will not fail. It is not that God does not offer His love; it is that I find myself unable to receive it. It is there, but I cannot accept that it is available to me in reality—because I conceive of myself as unlovable.

Deep down, I desire to be loved. But since I cannot believe this is possible, what I can and do experience instead is being needed and/ or being wanted. Encounters or relationships where I feel needed or wanted provide me with the intense experiences that are as close to being loved as I am likely to get—or maybe, having experienced nothing better, I do not even know that there *is* a love greater than these. Because of this, these encounters or relationships are powerful experiences that I want to repeat. I feel fleetingly in that moment that perhaps I could be loved—though this feeling cannot survive my cognitive scrutiny, which feels logical and objective even though it is actually constructed from my relational and emotional experience.

But St. Porphyrios warns us about seeking to be loved.[4] Rather, he says, we should love others, and it is up to them whether they love us. Sometimes I may love another only because I want them to love me back, but this is not the Christlike love the saint speaks of. Or I may imagine that I love another when I am actually just feeling some

---

4   Yiannitsiotis, *With Elder Porphyrios*, 47.

of the intensity of the love they are directing at me. And of course, even though I may seek some substitute for love in pornography, it is the last place I can find love and connection because I remain unseen, and therefore, unloved. But I want to be loved. I enjoy being loved—it is such a warm feeling. I do, in truth, need to be loved—I was created to be loved and always will be loved by God. I may even believe that God loves me, but this may still feel abstract. I feel the need for a physical manifestation of love so that I can believe in my heart that I am loved, as opposed to in my mind alone.

Because I need to be loved and am desperately afraid of rejection, I make myself a mask. In my shame about myself, I decorate that mask with an image I think will be acceptable to others and that reflects the way I would like to be, myself. The mask's shiny surface layer presents an acceptably faced version of me, and it protects the vulnerable me, the ugly me, the cowering, terrified little-child me below. But ironically, of course, in my desperation to avoid rejection, I have hidden myself from love. I have made the acceptance of myself in all my vulnerabilities and difficulties impossible. Nobody—including myself—can see the real me anymore because of my mask.

The mask, after all, does not, in reality, protect my true self, which requires to be known. The mask hides my true self away from the possibility of the love I deeply need. It feels like a protection, because I am so ashamed, so vulnerable. It seems as though I can show the shiny surface of my painted mask to the world and relate through it, but the problem is that even if someone does love the outer mask, my shame will remind me that they only love me because they think the mask they see is the real me. Saint Gregory of Nyssa alludes to this when he warns, "We may end up unconsciously protecting somebody who we are not, and leave our true selves unguarded."[5] The shiny layer

---

5   From Homily 2 on the Song of Songs, translation as quoted in Cox, Campbell, and Fulford, *Medicine of the Person*, 88.

protects the base layer of shame, but the real me behind the mask is left unknown, unseen, and unloved.

As I start to understand the mask of shame and begin to be aware that there is a real me behind it, I may still be drawn to pornography. But in awareness that there is more to me than my mask, can I also look at the people portrayed in pornography, knowing something about how they might have ended up there, and begin to see them as real people too? Can I begin to see behind their masks and to understand the feelings of the abused and the prostituted because I share the powerful ongoing desire to be needed and wanted—because perhaps for them, as for me, these are the closest things I have to being loved?

This lack of love is truly a deep loss, and being wanted physically only provides a pale image of the reality of love. So, in my loneliness and loss, I turn to other ways of coping. I may try to mask this loss in many ways. I might turn to alcohol or drugs; I may throw myself further into acting out sexually; I may throw myself into work or achievement; I may lose myself in depression and inertia. Through all these things, as I experience being essentially cut off from God, from creation, and from others, I seek the solution somehow in myself—or in what I put into myself. But the solution, of course, is not there—at least, it is not so near the surface of myself as all that. All these coping strategies build and decorate the masks over my real face, and they only serve to increase my feelings of shame. And in all these ways of coping, I am still attempting to maintain power and control over my life in the face of the underlying knowledge that power and control are precisely what I have lost. This is why the first step in twelve-step programs is the honest admission that I am powerless.

These attempts to cope, to fill the emptiness that comes when I feel unloved or unlovable, are all on the surface, and my surface is a lie, because it is a mask. In order to truly find love and to move beyond my shame, I need to go far deeper inside myself, through the nous, the eye of the heart, the deepest part of me, where I will begin to discern the image of God in all its beauty and the essential union with God that gives and sustains all life. The only way out of my destructive pattern of life is to find a way to turn to God, to grieve for all I have lost, and to get back onto the path of a life of repentance.

The first of St. Theophan's spiritual weapons in *Unseen Warfare* is "Never rely on yourself in anything."[6] When I attempt to control my own life and deal with my difficulties and struggles in myself, relying on myself is precisely what I am doing. I may have no confidence in my own abilities and may even try to give my life away to others for them to control. Nevertheless, if I look deep inside, I will probably find that even this is an attempt to control my own destiny, to work out my struggles under my own strength, to avoid the essential unknowing of life. When I do this, I give myself over to fear and despair rather than love.

"Never rely on yourself in anything" has a certain similarity to the first step of the twelve-step programs mentioned above: "We admitted we were powerless over our addiction—that our lives had become unmanageable."[7] However I express it, the first step when turning back to God—the first step of healing—is this admission: I am powerless under my own steam. I have been powerless for a long time. Admitting this is the prerequisite for a wholehearted turn to God, the source of life and the source of recovery from the effects of sexual sin in my life. It is a vitally important step, and with it I deeply accept my vulnerability and my need for real communion and active help. I admit that I am out of control. My attempts to direct my life, my attempts to follow my own desires or my own fears, these gave the

---

6   Theophan, *Unseen Warfare*, 81.
7   This is now the version of the first step as it appears in the "Big Book" in common use among AA twelve-step programs, which replaces the original version's "alcohol" with "our addiction." Alcoholics Anonymous, *Alcoholics Anonymous: The Story*, 59.

illusion of control—so this first step is to admit that those attempts were only an illusion—a mask. To admit this is to step into reality—to accept reality: I cannot give myself life. God created us, and we can only draw breath if He provides the life to do it.

This step is also an admission that in the way I have been reacting to my sexual desires, experiences, or abuse, I have been keeping something back for myself and/or from myself. I have been holding onto whatever it is I am using to fill the emptiness. Perhaps I am too ashamed to allow my loss or my emptiness to be seen—but even this shows me that I am still trying to maintain power over my own life, still holding my life hostage behind a mask of shame.

This first step is accepting reality, coming to myself like the prodigal son sitting among the pigs (Luke 15:11–32). With him I can reflect on where my life has led me under my own direction apart from God. He sits, wondering if he can eat the food of the pigs for sustenance because he has nothing else; I sit, looking at the dregs of life, desiring to fill myself with even the most unpleasant things because I am so empty that anything that can fill me may seem worth a try. When I am at the point that I finally do see the emptiness of this kind of life, it helps me to surrender to reality—and in making contact with reality, I am beginning to dismantle my masks of shame. As those masks lose their power, it becomes easier to see my other kinds of masks and begin to remove those too. At this point I am no longer trying to fight off reality with my desires or fears, and I recognize that the ground of all reality is God. I recognize that I had been using my habits and patterns of life to avoid coming before God, to avoid coming before ultimate Reality. And when I admit my powerlessness, I admit that I have been refusing to deal with reality and that *now* is the favorable time to start.

Well-intentioned others may even try to stop me from admitting my own powerlessness—either out of fear for where it might lead me, or perhaps because they have come to depend on the version of me they know—the shiny surface of my mask. But in truth it is a relief when I surrender this mask, this false life that I have been calling my own and trying to manage on my own. I have received life as a gift from God, and I must return it to Him, for the one who loses his life for Christ's sake gains it (Matt. 16:25). It is His and it is also mine—but it is most mine when I return it to Christ to find out who I truly am and what this beautiful gift will bring. Because whatever I may believe or feel, my life is in truth a beautiful gift from God, given in love and reflecting God's own beauty.

Sometimes my shame makes it hard to see life that way. Sometimes my life seems more like a curse. Sometimes I don't want to hold onto it, and it seems as if losing it—giving it away or even throwing it away—is the best option. But rather than throw it away, I can give it back to the one who gave it to me. And as I begin this journey of returning my self to God, like the prodigal setting out on the journey back to his father's house, I also find that this is the beginning of my participation in the life of Christ, voluntarily ascending with Him to the Cross. This is where I learn—with Him and in Him—to give up my attempts in power and control to own my life. As I begin to practice this, though the journey may be rocky at first, with many twists and turns, I begin to find that I can trust Christ. However much others have failed me when I have trusted them, Christ is perfectly trustworthy and will never abandon me. Equally, He will never force me to turn to Him: He will love me in perfect freedom and in total respect of my freedom. This is the kind of love I need to receive and to learn to give. There is no other way but to surrender to Him.

Yet even surrendering the ugly in me is so hard it can seem impossible. Sometimes it seems easier to surrender what is most beautiful. All addiction in the end is the unwilling but inevitable preference to surrender the most beautiful over the ugliest as I choose my "drug" of choice over what I truly desire. But Christ loves me with an abundant, life-giving love: all the good that I surrender to Him He will return in abundance, and in His love, all that is ugly He will transform into beauty.

My surrender to God, my admission of powerlessness, my admission that I cannot truly rely on myself: these align me with reality, with truth. These put me in touch with life as it really is, and this is a step away from masks of shame and into humility. The admission of powerlessness is also important, because it enables me to seek help from others rather than going it alone. But it is actually this other aspect of the step that is at the heart of why the step is so significant—it is a step into humility, which enables me to make contact with Truth.

To live in Truth (to find communion with God) is to jettison the masks. It is this taste of communion as I surrender to God that enables me to give up those things I have depended on to protect me. I begin to surrender those parts of myself that are the root of my struggles: my habits, my patterns of life, my memories, my relationships . . . everything. In order to understand what it truly means to love in a Godlike way, I need to prepare myself to surrender everything. Especially when I believe my life is worthless—but even if I value it—I may be willing to lay down my life for my friends. But could I ever be ready to sacrifice what is most precious to me, what I care about protecting most? What about the life of my child? Of course, God will not demand this of me—only God Himself would be able to make such a sacrifice. He will provide the ram for the sacrifice in place of Isaac (Gen. 22). But the question is important nonetheless, because if I am not willing to prepare the offering as Abraham did and as the Theotokos did, I am still holding something back.

And as long as I hold anything back behind my mask, I am still primarily attempting to preserve my own life in my own way. But this will only cause me to lose it. Only when I give up the life I have created will I have the chance of saving the life God has given me (Luke 17:33). When I admit my powerlessness, I begin to lift the mask and align myself with truth and unknowing, and I learn to surrender everything—including my habits, my needs, my addictions. I surrender them to healing love.

The reality of being loved is far different from the delusions of pornography and its pornographic images of shame on my masks. When we love and are loved, we will experience mutual and genuine interest in each other as real persons, as whole persons. We will accept the whole of one another and be accepted just as we are, including all we do not like in ourselves. We may find ourselves beginning to change for the better because of this. One who truly loves us will be able to see some of our characteristic behaviors and expressions as endearing rather than irritating (this is the sense in which beauty is in the eye of the beholder—it is not about beauty so much as the ability to love). We will begin to share a genuine interest in each other's feelings and experiences, simply because those are all part of us and for no other reason. We will learn to see deeply into each other beyond the mask, beyond the toughened scars on our surface, and into the vulnerability that lies beneath. We will begin to see beyond the smile when one of us is weeping internally, and beyond the outer stillness when there is merriment or deep joy beneath. We will find that shame is overcome, that love and life are more powerful than delusion and death.

Of course, in this earthly life, this vision of love without the mask will never be fully and permanently realized, but can we begin to offer this vision to others? And can we find the heart to offer it precisely because we know what life behind the masks is like?

A Prayer of Saint Nikolaj of Žiča[8]

Deliver my soul from self-delusion, my God,
so that my body may also be delivered from bodily sin.

---

8   Velimirovich, *Prayers*, 137.

CHAPTER 6

Fantasy: The Mockery of God

LIKE THE SHADOWY LAYERS OF lust and shame on my masks, fantasy is designed to protect me from the dangers of reality—or at least create for me a more palatable version of reality—but has the effect of cutting me off from the possibility of real relationship. *Fantasy* is defined in English as "the faculty or activity of imagining impossible or improbable things," or as "an idea with no basis in reality" (OED). And *imagining*, in turn, means creating a mental image, or believing in something that has no basis in reality. While our society does see fantasy as having no basis in reality, this is somewhat misleading for a variety of reasons. The first reason is that, as I have already said, nothing can exist that has no basis in God, who is ultimate Reality. This applies just as much to ideas, thoughts, feelings, and relationships as it does to the physical. Another reason is that since the fantasy takes place in my own mind, *I* am the basis of that reality which the fantasy connects to. If we are thinking iconologically, it is also apparent that all fantasy has meaning. I create the fantasy for a reason, and the way the fantasy takes form will, if seen iconologically, tell me something about the deeper needs and distortions I am experiencing within.

Despite the definition's reference to unreality, in modern Western culture we tend to use the word *imagination* positively—and to use the word *fantasy* either positively or negatively. Yet, if we explore the writings of the Church Fathers, we will find that they use these terms in almost universally negative contexts. This shocks our modern sensibility because we have a neo-Romantic tendency to glorify the individual imagination and self-expression.

Why do the concepts of imagination and fantasy have such negative connotations in the ascetic literature of the Church? One reason I have already mentioned has to do with the danger of creating an image that tempts us away from our focus on God, either because it causes us to objectify or idolize our own creation, or because it is a conduit to the demonic rather than the divine world. A second, related reason might be that the ascetic Fathers in their spiritual maturity have in mind pure prayer, or imageless prayer. And at this point, the Church Fathers tell us, any image—no matter how good in itself—becomes a distraction from the imageless communion with God experienced in pure prayer. Pure prayer anticipates that day when we no longer need to "see through a glass, darkly" as St. Paul puts it (in the well-known KJV translation of 1 Cor. 13:12).[1] In this world, we can see directly only shadows and veils, icons and images, that lead us in faith to perceive what is beyond this world. But in the last day, in eschatological fullness, we will no longer "see through a glass, darkly"; we will see "face to face." Similarly, we might keep a photo of a loved one close in his or her absence. We may even kiss it, but when the loved one is present, our focus is on him or her in person. In the meantime, the icon is, according to the hymns from Vespers for the Sunday of Orthodoxy, both the safeguard of the Orthodox faith and a source of healing.

---

1   Note that "glass" refers to a mirror. The Greek phrase here translated "darkly" is ἐν αἰνίγματι, literally, *in an enigma*.

In this light, the dangers of creating a mental image are obvious, given all we have seen about the nature of imagery and the iconographic or pornographic understandings of the physical world. As to whether any given case of a mental image is good or not, surely it depends firstly on whether we are aware that the image points at something or someone beyond itself, and secondly on what it is pointing toward—what its prototype is. Imagination in the sense of creativity is not necessarily pornographic; as human beings, we are not only creative, we are co-creators with God in all that we do—but we can use that God-given creative power either for good or for bad. The same argument applies to fantasy. The genre of fiction we call *fantasy* includes C. S. Lewis's *Narnia* series and Tolkien's *Lord of the Rings*, and these authors use fantasy and imaginary situations as veils to reveal a deeper vision of truth or meaning. Whether a particular imaginative work is good depends on how true—how much in accord with ultimate Reality—its deeper meaning is. So as co-creators who are fallen creatures, we can use our creativity in cooperation with God's creative power, or we can use it apart from God.

Imagination is after all a capacity of the soul, and therefore a reflection of the image of God in us. Like all the capacities of the soul, we can use it to grow closer to God (as a veil that outlines what lies beyond) or to create a barrier (a mask) in front of the face of God, which blocks our relationship. In other words, we can use imagination to aim for the target (God), but it can "miss the mark" (be sinful). It can be a part of developing my love of God and neighbor (including my enemies!) or a path that leads me away from myself and my ability to truly relate, by inflaming and exercising my passions. In awareness that we can use imagination positively or negatively, let us have a closer look at some of the dangers of imagination and fantasy in general.

Saint John Climacus describes fantasy in this way: "Fantasy is the deception of the eyes when the nous is asleep. Fantasy is a displacement of the nous when the body is awake. Fantasy is a vision of something non-existent."[2] The nous, the "eye of the heart," we might describe as the organ of iconographic seeing and iconological understanding. The nous is the center of our soul, or heart, the point at which we can connect most directly to God—which is also to say, connect with ultimate reality. If imagination or fantasy fills my nous, I end up focused on what is unreal, miss the mark of what is real, and thereby cut myself off from God at my root.

Much fantasy about relationships, sexual or otherwise, is like this. To fantasize about someone is to fail to see the person *as* a person. Just as in pornography, when I fantasize, I objectify, fail to relate, and fail to love. I fail to give anything of myself; there is no real relationship. I see without being seen. In fact, when in fantasy I fail to see the other person as a real person, I am also failing to see myself as a real person, made for relationship, made to love and be loved forever. It is the opposite of venerating an icon. With an icon, as I have already said, I am the one who is seen—the reverse perspective of the icon means I am the one at the vanishing point of the perspective. I am seen through the window of the icon as the saint looks out at me from the vastness of eternity. But when I fantasize, I remain alone and unseen.

While icons bind me to ultimate truth and Reality, fantasy's grasp on reality is tenuous. Fantasy starts with reality and begins to create a vision of something based on that reality but modified toward my desires in a way that is improbable or unlikely to really happen. As it progresses, it can quickly become an idea with an ever-shrinking basis in reality—closer and closer to total nonexistence. The more I fantasize, the more I base my fantasy images on previous fantasy, and the less connection they have with reality. As I practice relating

---

2   Climacus, *Ladder*, from step 3. My own translation from the Greek text
     online: https://el.wikisource.org/wiki/Κλίμαξ. (An alternative translation
     can be found at Climacus, 19.)

to people in fantasy instead of in reality, and as I spend more time in my fantasy, I decrease both my ability and my opportunity to relate to another real person. Spending time fantasizing, then, reduces both the opportunity for communion and the ability to participate in it. Venerating an icon has the opposite effect: to venerate is to imagine—in the sense of bringing something to mind—something of the ultimate Reality that is beyond our senses. An icon makes what it portrays really present; it reveals what might otherwise be outside the ability of the senses to perceive. A fantasy, on the other hand, substitutes for reality: it is the painted layer on a mask that misdirects and obscures rather than revealing.

Sexual fantasy, in particular, is pornography of the mind. And just as with pornography, this is sexual abuse. Christ said that just to look at another woman with lust is to commit adultery with her (Matt. 5). This happens without her consent, so it is not too strong to say that to sexually fantasize about a woman, or any other person, is to rape her in my heart, and likewise, to look at a pornographic image or video of another person is to rape her in my heart. Fantasy, like pornography, is violence and theft, and it leaves the person who has become an object violated.

Therefore, when I fantasize, I not only avoid the relationship I desire, I abuse the person I desire. Moreover, in doing so, I build these aspects of behavior into my character and person. Recent neurological studies have demonstrated this, finding that imagining something has a very similar effect on the brain to actually experiencing it, because "everything your 'immaterial' mind imagines leaves material traces."[3] Because of this, it is bad advice to tell people with vio-

---

3   Doidge, *Brain That Changes* 232. See the whole chapter on imagination in
     Doidge, 215–233. One example the text gives is an experiment that taught
     people to play a simple tune on the piano. It compared a group learning
     physically with a group learning only in their imagination without touching
     a physical piano keyboard. "Remarkably, mental practice alone produced

lent or destructive sexual desires that to fantasize is good, with the idea it will make them less likely to act their fantasies out. In reality, fantasizing about something not only increases the desire for it and opens the spirit to the possibility of doing it, it even lays patterns in the brain that increase not only the expectation of experiencing it but even the ability to do it. Where possible, I should avoid even thinking about fantasies I have had. As St. John Climacus advises, "Let no one get into the habit of thinking over during the daytime the phantasies that have occurred to him during sleep; for the aim of the demons in prompting this is to defile us while we are awake by making us think about our dreams."[4]

In fact, there is plenty of evidence showing that fantasy and pornography can so capture a person in spirit, mind, and body that they end up preferring their perfectly tailored fantasy to messy reality. A young man heavily into animated porn illustrated just how far this can go when he commented that animated porn characters are "less disgusting . . . (and cleaner) than real women."[5] But this preference for lonely fantasy over a real relationship is only the beginning of the ways in which fantasy (including pornography) "kills love."[6] It takes away the ability to be attentive, it swallows the hours, it breaks communication and connection, and it ultimately destroys relationships. Fantasy is all about avoidance, and in one sense it delivers—if I ask to be left alone often enough, in the end, I will be. My avoidance will be complete and forever. However, in another sense, it will fail, because ultimately, one thing I am trying to avoid is my own real experience. In escapism, I am trying to prevent having to live with my own

---

the same physical changes in the motor system as actually playing the piece" (220).

4   Climacus, *Ladder*, 15:56, 112.

5   "'Real People Are Gross': 3 Reasons Why Animated Porn Is So Popular," *Fight the New Drug*, accessed July 30, 2022, https://fightthenewdrug.org /animated-porn-is-gaining-popularity/.

6   "Porn Kills Love" is a slogan of *Fight the New Drug*. They sell T-shirts!

thinking, having to be with myself, and having to face the reality of myself and my real situation. But I am the one thing I will never be able to escape. Wherever I try to escape to, whether it be a physical place or a mental one, I will still always be there.

Escapism—coping by avoidance—is strongly correlated with depression. Escapism not only manifests in fantasy; it can also manifest in social media use (when it is used as a substitute for real relationship), video streaming, and video gaming, as well as in drugs, gambling, and other activities and behaviors, whether or not they are in themselves unhealthy. Escapism creates a self-defeating vicious circle as it reduces my motivation to take action in real life, and in doing so, it throws me back to the fantasy. As I get caught in this loop of escapism, I retreat into fantasy again because I feel powerless. In my fantasy I am all-powerful—even if I do not think of myself that way as I fantasize. Godlike, I create worlds and people; godlike, I destroy them. But this is a mockery of God, for none of it connects to Reality, and therefore none of it can ultimately satisfy. For this fake godlikeness, I may end up forgoing the genuine Godlikeness that I am offered in Christ: "He, indeed, assumed humanity that we might become God."[7]

I have noted above that any repeated practice forms spiritual patterns and neurological pathways. This exercise of power in fantasy increases the objectification of the other more and more over time and can end up narrowing my vision so far that I lose the necessity or possibility of real relationship—and this literally destroys me as a *person*. It destroys my freedom and leaves me imprisoned behind my mask; my true face is lost in the fantasy. Alternatively, it can cause me to focus on the objectified fact rather than the person. The ultimate end of this path is that I would be conditioned so thoroughly in the practice of objectification that even when faced with a real human

---

7   Athanasius, *On the Incarnation*, 93.

person, I would overlook that personal reality and see and treat a human being as a physical object. This is not an exaggeration: it is visibly the case in much modern pornography, and it is the lived experience of some people who have been raped.

These destructive kinds of fantasies do not have to be sexual to be pornographic. As I have said before, anything that takes a part of creation that is meant to be iconographic (a writing about God) and separates it from its root in the ultimate Reality of God is creating an obscene writing (a pornography). It might be a fantasy about becoming rich—winning the lottery, for example. Or a fantasy about becoming extremely witty in order to put down someone who has offended me. Yet another kind of fantasy is imagining I have reached a plane of holiness I have not: trying to imitate Christ or the saints outwardly without living into their likeness. Of such conduct Dr. Johnson once said, "Almost all absurdity of conduct arises from the imitation of those whom we cannot resemble."[8]

Indeed, while I may take any of my fantasies very seriously— they are, after all, however misguided, attempts to meet deep, real needs within—to others they may seem absurd, and rightly so, for they address themselves to needs they cannot really fulfill. But how do I avoid fantasizing in this negative, anti-iconographic way? One important piece of advice many ascetic Fathers have repeated throughout history is that I need to cut off such an intrusive thought at the root. Saint Paisios described these intrusive thoughts or images as being like airplanes circling around: the key thing is not to let them land.[9] Even to entertain such a thought or image for a second gives it entry into the nous.

The easiest time to act is always now, never later. So as soon as the image appears, I can make the sign of the cross and invite the presence

---

8   Johnson, *The Rambler*, Reference no. 135, 372. (Note: This volume contains numbers 71–140.)

9   Aggeloglou, *Elder Paisios*, 29–30.

of Christ into my heart. When Christ Himself was tempted in the wilderness by intrusive thoughts from the devil, He referred at once to the presence of God, using quotations from Scripture (Matt. 4:1–11). Since fantasy is often a symptom or a symbol of personal isolation—of being in the wilderness—this invocation of God's presence through the words of Scripture, prayer, or the sign of the cross is one way I can address it. I can also engage with reality through God's creation. I might make contact with real people, either in person or by phone or chat, or I might go for a walk in nature. Alongside this, at such a moment it is opportune to arrange a time for confession.

It is important to acknowledge that my misdirected desires will often create the opportunity for fantasies to arise, so I should be ready for them. Without dwelling on them, I can be aware of what my particular fantasies and daydreams tend to be, and whether they really bring me closer to union with Christ or rather move me further away. And when I catch myself falling into a fantasy or daydream of this type, I can try inviting Christ in and letting His light fill the darkness in my soul.

A Prayer of Light[10]

O Christ, the True Light,
Who enlightens and sanctifies everyone that comes into the world:
let the light of Your countenance be signed upon us,
that in it we may behold the unapproachable light,
and guide our steps into the way of Your commandments,
by the intercessions of Your all-holy Mother and of all Your saints.

---

10   Prayer of the first hour, a modern-language version of that found in *Book of Hours*, 70.

CHAPTER 7

Behind Our Masks

W E HAVE SEEN WITH OUR lust, shame, and fantasy masks
that everything we find behind the mask, however distress-
ing, is a sign of life that has the potential to be shared, authentic, interpersonal life—a potential the masks obscure. If I do not take steps to
live that more real life, in the end the mask will be the only thing I
have left, and there will be nothing behind it for anyone to find. C. S.
Lewis's book *The Great Divorce* (of heaven and hell) illustrates this
in the most dramatic way, when the Tragedian, the character-mask
an ordinary man uses to protect his true self, in the end swallows up
the real man and becomes his gravestone and epitaph: a dead—if
dramatic—shell, a meaningless actor with no play to perform.

Father Pavel Florensky, priest, scientist, and martyr, in his book
Iconostasis, also speaks of this loss of the person behind the mask:

> When a face has become a mask, we can know nothing whatever
> about what Kant would call its *noumenon* [that is, its true reality as
> opposed to what can be perceived]; neither can we (with the positiv-
> ists) find any reason at all to affirm the real existence of that face. For
> (using the Apostle's phrase) "having their conscience seared," these
> mask-faces are dark: not one single ray from God's image within

them reaches the surface of their personality: and so we cannot know whether or not God's judgement has been wholly accomplished in them and that they have had taken away from them the token, or covenant, in them which is God's image.[1]

The reality of the person behind the mask is hidden from life, and the more it is hidden, the less we can tell whether the real person still exists behind it. The mask increasingly obscures the image of God within us and prevents us from being seen face to face. What we do know is that while life is still present, the image is still present, however far it is from the surface—however thick the mask. Only at our death will those who see our mask have the uncertainty Fr. Pavel refers to, as to whether the real person lives on.

In the end, however, we do not have the power in this life to create the fully convincing, totally effective mask Fr. Pavel alludes to, though our masks will fool some. In C. S. Lewis's story mentioned above, the Tragedian-mask did not fool the man's wife. She would not speak to the Tragedian, only to the real man himself—even when he was barely perceptible, his reality fading away as he ceded more and more of himself to the mask. Even the mask turns out to be to some extent translucent, and it becomes—at least when viewed by perceptive, compassionate, purified eyes—partly a veil. And we cannot escape, even in our fallen and sinful creativity, the image of God in us that communicates truth. Everything we paint on the mask turns out also to have a deeper meaning, and by following the symbolism—by seeing iconologically—we can come to greater self-knowledge.

Pornography may be anti-iconographic, but every desire for pornography, just like every mask, still inevitably reflects the essential nature of the world, since evil cannot create anything—it can only

---

1   Florensky, *Iconostasis*, 56.

twist and misshape what is good in creation. So if I am aware of what I am consuming, I can see what patterns my relationships and encounters have formed in me. I might see patterns relating to my past or childhood experiences, my family background, and important relationships. For example, if I have suffered from abuse, I may detach myself from any feelings of anger or aggression, as I can associate these only with the hurt others inflicted on me. The shiny surface of my mask will be a picture of gentleness and compassion, while the shadowy layer below will be the anger and aggression locked inside, which may express itself in unpredictable and uncontrolled ways.

Trauma of various kinds is often central to the creation of masks—and it does not need to be "objectively" major trauma. The context, intensity, amount of time, and number of repetitions are all relevant, but the central question is what effect the traumatic experience or experiences have had on me. Especially as a child, I was very vulnerable. But even as an adult, I am still vulnerable, no matter how deeply I try to hide my vulnerability or how many shields and defenses I set up against it in my masks. And my masks do not protect me well enough: I am still hurt. My despair is existential because the layers of my masks cut off my real self from any true encounter.

There are two ways to move beyond this existential separation, this hiddenness behind the mask. I can learn to slowly lift the mask and begin to reveal what is beneath, or someone else can find a way to see beyond the mask and begin to perceive the truer me inside. In practice, both of these need to work together, as without a loving other, how can I learn to trust enough to reveal myself? And if another does start to see beyond the mask, unless I can trust them enough to begin to reveal myself in response, the light they start to shine behind the mask will be painful and terrifying.

With the right way of seeing, the mask becomes translucent—it begins to appear as a veil that reveals the outline of what is below. But if I hide behind my mask and persist in requiring others to relate to it instead of to the real me, my reality will fade, as we saw above in the case of the Tragedian. As we have also seen, a purified eye—an eye of compassion and the holy desire for communion—will have some ability to see through my masks.

But there is another kind of perceptive eye that can detect at least the existence of the mask and perceive that something more real lies behind it. That is the eye of acquisitive desire. This is what can happen in cases of grooming, which leads to sexual or other abuse: I am drawn in as a victim because I feel that someone has seen the real me behind the mask. I feel that finally I have been seen, that now I will be heard, that there is the potential of real connection if I allow myself to step out from behind my mask. When someone abuses this vulnerability I have revealed, of course, I reapply the mask with all the more determination. I suffer behind it, still unable to destroy my human need for connection but even more hopeless about the possibility of attaining it.

An experience one woman had while in prostitution illustrates such a determined reapplication of her mask:

> I remember one man in particular because he didn't seem interested in taking explicit photographs; this was unusual. He told me to pose any way I wanted and never instructed that I take my clothes off. I remember sitting balanced in the window ledge, with my head resting against the wall and my chin tilted up and closing my eyes as though I was deep in thought, and suddenly I was deep in thought, and I was imagining that I was a model; that it had all worked out in the modeling agency and I was just doing a day's work. The click of his camera brought me back. He told me that it would be a very beautiful photograph. I felt injured; violated in a new way. He had caught something

of the real me on his roll of film. That was a new sort of lesson in never letting your guard down.[2]

This is a tragic description of a failed attempt at real encounter and the degree to which we may fear connection (in many cases with good reason). There seems to be a movement here in a positive, personal direction, but by a man whose motivation is unclear, so the encounter causes the woman to further withdraw behind her mask. She makes the mask of protection indiscriminate because she has learned that danger can come from anywhere, and what appear to be sheep may in fact be wolves behind a sheep's mask. This context is too dangerous for her to believe the hints of authenticity.

What I need for myself, then, in order to feel safe when I reveal what is behind the mask—and what I need to provide for others— is a relationship of safety and genuine compassion, wherein I can show my vulnerabilities and the other person will not take advantage of me. Where I can learn to reveal myself, in confidence that in this reality I will not be destroyed. In such a relationship, I can allow my mask to soften into a veil. Rather than obscuring my real features, the veil provides a cover of modesty, but through the veil I can be seen. Rather than the hard boundary wall of the mask, which locks me inside, it is a semi-permeable boundary enabling me to maintain my safety and dignity, and yet allowing me to be seen, to encounter, and to relate. In this world, the veil is our means of connection, and thus the icon is a type of veil that enables us to see and relate to the truth of spiritual reality beyond the world that is immediately available to our physical senses.

It is clear that our need to relate, to connect, to know and be known personally means that we have to come out from behind our masks and reveal ourselves. However, once something that was

---

2   Moran, *Paid For*, 72.

previously hidden is revealed, there are consequences—positive and negative—whether we immediately see them or not. When we begin to reveal ourselves, it is automatically a confession. And as soon as we start talking about anything—and most of all, if we speak about ourselves—we create the possibility of actions in ourselves and others that we might not have predicted.

Going back to the very beginning, we see Adam and Eve in the Garden playing out these intended and unintended, predictable and unpredictable, positive and negative consequences. The evil one manipulated the revelation of the significance of the Tree of the Knowledge of Good and Evil, with the result that we continue to fall into sin and separation from each other and from God. And the other side of the coin is that God continues to work and to find ways of using our very separation and sin as a means of teaching us freedom and love.

As with every revelation, every move to see behind masks and veils in this fallen world is a double-edged sword. We can see this in Western society as, for at least the last century or two, our society has been in a gradual process of opening up discussions of sex, sexuality, and gender. Many people view this precisely as opening up human freedom and love. This is partly true because, on the one hand, the ability to open up and discuss our deepest feelings, temptations, and desires enables us to loosen our masks and thereby enables deeper connection and true intimacy, so that we may find fuller communion with each other and with God. And freedom to discuss our desires may be liberating not necessarily in the sense (most common today) that by doing so we are free to act on them without public censure, but in the sense that opening up the darkest corners of our hearts enables light to shine in—the true Light, the Light of Christ. But on the other hand, such revelation can be dangerous. We have already looked at the possibility of being taken advantage of when we start to reveal ourselves. The other possible misuse of our openness is that our experiences and our descriptions of them may arouse misdirected and distorted desires in others.

In the Orthodox Church, we do, of course, have the Mystery of Confession, which provides a way for us to begin opening up our dark corners in the presence of a confessor—a confessor who is hopefully loving enough to show us total acceptance, and also discerning enough to help us see what in us does not reflect the image of God. Through this, the confessor can help us move toward acquiring a greater likeness of God. But for many of us, this relatively closed and protected environment does not seem to be enough. In the early Church, of course, people often made such confessions in front of the congregation. And as we read in *The Ladder*, St. John Climacus describes an example of this even in his time (the sixth and seventh centuries), when a novice was encouraged to give his confession before the whole assembly of the brotherhood for the edification of all.[3]

This public confession would of course have been humiliating to deliver. And I would certainly never choose public humiliation! But sometimes if I have been publicly humiliated, the result can be a tremendous sense of release—my shame has been revealed, and therefore its power has been neutralized. Particularly in the case of sexual temptations and sins, and particularly if I feel condemned by my awareness of an existing strong aversion to my feelings and experiences among the people around me, I have a very great sense of shame. Not a healthy shame, but a toxic shame that closes me in on myself and prevents me from finding a way to that very vulnerability that is necessary for developing deep, loving relationships. And so I come to feel very strongly that I do not want to continue to sweep my sins under the carpet. I feel, in the modern way of speaking, that I want to "come out of the closet." I feel the need to reveal things about myself that will humble and yet also free me in the eyes of my

---

3   Climacus, *Ladder*, 4:11–12, 23–25.

brethren, and that will provide the opportunity for true vulnerability on both sides. Whether I am able to do this by choice, or whether it happens for other reasons, as I am exposed in front of my fellows, and as they have to find a way to deal with such a revelation, true vulnerability (on both sides) can lead to a deeper, more real relationship of love. This was behind the confession of the penitent in *The Ladder*. Saint John Climacus asked the abbot why he had asked the penitent to do this, and the abbot answered that it was, first, "to deliver [him] from future shame by present shame" and second, to encourage others to have the same freedom to confess their hidden sins and thereby receive forgiveness.[4]

There is freedom in confession, in being able to be open and share my struggles. But as I said above, in this fallen world, the consequences of revelation are not only positive but also negative. As we lay out more and more of these kinds of issues openly in the public square, we influence the thoughts and feelings of others. Those inchoate longings that we sense inside but have found no way to express may start to hang themselves on the thoughts and desires of others. This happens because we learn to categorize our feelings, and even ourselves, according to what we learn from others.

There is strong evidence of this exact thing happening in pornography. On the one hand, pornography reflects the desires and fetishes of porn users. But on the other hand, it also forms them. Porn sites immediately confront visitors with suggestions of desires and fetishes they have probably never thought of before and which may not interest them at first. But as I said above, fantasy tends to build on fantasy. This parallels the process of toleration in addiction, as the addict requires more and more intense experiences to deliver the same feeling. Thus habitual users of porn will sometimes stray into more and more specific and peculiar, and often violently abusive, fantasy

---

4   Climacus, *Ladder*, 4:12, 24–25.

worlds.[5] As porn sites continue to build data on the patterns of users, they become ever cleverer in suggesting the next new fetish to each viewer. Thus, the revelation of one person's fetishistic desire becomes a new temptation for thousands, if not millions more. We can also see this same pattern in the changing face of sexual relationships. It is undeniably true that sexual practices have changed quite dramatically over the last few decades, and practices that were previously very rare—including risky and potentially harmful practices—have become commonplace.[6] The revelation of one person's desire again may become a temptation for many.

It is an open question whether the dangers outweigh the rewards in this new openness. But certainly, every revelation comes with great responsibility, and our society currently does not appear to recognize the existence of this responsibility, let alone take it seriously. We need to learn that more knowledge about things is not in itself good; it all depends on how we use it. There again, we cannot sweep everything back under the carpet, and so we have to learn how best to deal with what has been revealed to us. There can, however, be no general rule about whether we speak openly about our struggles, how openly, and in what context. Each of us needs to reflect carefully on these matters and discuss them with trusted spiritual guides and wise confessors. And when we decide to lift the mask and speak out, we need to be ready to face all the potential consequences. Given the

---

5   There are many reports of such experiences, along with descriptions of the addictive process, in Wilson, *Your Brain on Porn*. See also Mikkola, *Pornography*, 46; Paul, *Pornified*, 81, 86–92, 227–229.

6   See, for example Flood, "Pornography, violence," Chapter 11; Boyle, *Everyday Pornography*, 170–171; Debby Herbenick et al., "Frequency, Method, Intensity, and Health Sequelae of Sexual Choking Among U.S. Undergraduate and Graduate Students," *Archives of Sexual Behavior* 51(2022): 3121–3139; Lewis et al., "Heterosexual Practices among Young People in Britain: Evidence from Three National Surveys of Sexual Attitudes and Lifestyles," *Journal of Adolescent Health* 61, no. 6 (December 2017): 694–702.

much greater openness within our society on these issues, we are all now faced with some of the responsibility of the confessor: when these revelations appear before us, we will need to be ready to love and accept the person as he or she is and yet also exercise discernment and help to shine the Light of Christ into every dark place. This is why being prepared by thinking about these issues in advance is so important to all of us.

So once I have reached the place where I want to begin to lift my mask and share something of my personal desires and struggles, the question is, how do I express myself? What do I say and what do I not say, and what is the basis for these decisions? The story of St. Mary of Egypt can help me answer these questions, whether I am telling my own story or listening to someone else's. When the holy priest and hermit St. Zosimas asks St. Mary of Egypt (the former harlot at that point living a life of holiness in the desert) to tell him her story, she wonders aloud whether she will defile him by speaking of it. But he wants to learn from her. She describes her story as her "shame," yet he describes it as "an edifying story."[7] There are some important aspects of the way she tells her story that can be a model for me when I tell mine.

Saint Mary starts with humility. She sees her shame, is aware that her life needs to change: she perceives the need for repentance very clearly. It is only in the light of this clarity that her story will be a true revelation, a true lifting of the mask rather than the creation of a new one. She tells her story carefully, focusing on the mercy she received and with gratitude for her blessings, and in constant awareness of the potential impact of the story both on herself and on St. Zosimas. She is uncompromising and specific about the things she did and what had happened to her, but without any details that could titillate or cause the sort of inverted pride that would create a new mask. And

---

7   Thekla, *Great Canon*, 122.

likewise, she shows no pride in having overcome her established sins but gives all glory to God.

Saint Mary of Egypt at this point was clearly partaking of the divine life inasmuch as that is possible while still in the earthly body. Although she expressed doubts in herself and about whether or not to reveal her past to St. Zosimas, she clearly had great discernment, and it was undoubtedly, as St. Zosimas said, an edifying story. I have less confidence in my own discernment, so I will be careful about when, to whom, and how to communicate my story—careful, but not avoidant. I wish to take off the mask, but I know I have no choice but to retain the veil, because it is not possible for me in this earthly life to communicate fully in truth, face to face. My words are themselves a veil, and what others see through them depends not only on my own limited ability to communicate appropriately but also on the hearer, and on your eyes, the eye of your heart, unknown reader.

Reflecting on stories such as that of St. Mary of Egypt, which is read in church every year during Lent, is one way we can connect to the stories that lie within ourselves and begin to learn about what lies behind our masks. They help us start to put our innermost realities into stories ourselves: into words, pictures, or music. We can begin to find our own ways of communicating our truer selves so that we can be seen as through a veil, rather than remaining hidden behind a mask.

When I am telling my own story, it can sometimes be difficult for me to know to what extent I am revealing a true story of the real me emerging from behind the mask and to what extent I am still telling a story of the masks I have created. To help with this, it is useful to have other perspectives on my life, past and present, and bring them into conversation with my own current narrative. One way of doing this is through being attentive to other people who know me. Another way is through using a journal. If I record my reflections, thoughts, and prayers over time, my words in the past can connect me to an earlier version of myself, reminding me what I was doing and how I was thinking and feeling previously. Sometimes I read back some part of my journal and find a contradiction there to the version of the story that I tell now. Likewise, people I know well may remember things differently from the way I remember them. These cases provide further opportunities for self-discovery. For example, I may see that one of these versions comes from one of my masks or one of its layers. If it does not seem to be connected to my masks, I may be able to discern what is communicated by the difference between the way I understood myself and my behavior in the past and the way I describe it now.

One former prostitute alludes to this kind of difference when she notes the contrast between the way women who are currently involved in prostitution tend to defend it and the way women who are no longer involved in prostitution often campaign to protect the women who remain:

> There are, of course, women in prostitution who'll defend it. Why wouldn't they? For many women in prostitution, this is all they've got; and who among us wouldn't defend the only thing we've got? . . . It's not just easier, while you're still being prostituted, to tell yourself that this is work. As a matter of psychological survival, it is simply emotionally necessary.[8]

This is why I have my masks—it is a matter of psychological survival. Until I find a better way, those masks are all I have. So if I am involved in prostitution, and I don't see the possibility of an alternative way to live, I need a story that enables me to believe I can manage it and live with it. The obvious story is that this way of living is

---

8 Rachel Moran, "The reality of prostitution is not complex. It is simple," *Psyche*, June 1, 2022, https://psyche.co/ideas/the-reality-of-prostitution-is-not -complex-it-is-simple.

all right, that I am choosing it, that I am even benefiting from it. But once I am freed from the necessity of that life, I am able to see it in a different light.

Continuing to hide behind the mask is in fact, in some circumstances, a matter of psychological survival. To come out from behind the mask while still in this situation would be suicide. A change of life must come first. What exactly this change will need to be will be different for each of us. It will involve some form of repentance and some form of transformation, but it may also require social, relational, geographical, or some other form of change. It will likely require some assistance from others, which means I may have to drop my mask a little and show my vulnerability, however dangerous that may seem. None of this is easy, and reaching this point may require a lifetime of work. Through the mercy of God, until we are in a place to start this process, we have the icon. Through the icon, the saints, the Mother of God, and Christ Himself can speak to us of the heavenly realities beyond this life. And they do not speak from a place of safety at a total remove from our earthly reality—each person we meet in an icon has lived through this earthly suffering and in the process has found their heavenly home.

When hiding behind the mask is "a matter of psychological survival," then what the mask covers is the abyss, the void, total existential despair. There is a risk that as soon as I begin to lift the mask and become aware of the abyss, I will quickly put my mask back—put my conventional self back together again. However, once I have glimpsed the abyss, it may be hard to believe in the reality of the mask as much as I did before. From this point—even if I am not yet ready to let go of the mask—I can perhaps peek into the abyss a little. It will keep me in touch with reality, even if I am not yet ready to live in it, in all its terrifying fullness. Saint Sophrony puts it this way: "Stand on the edge of the abyss and when you feel that it is beyond your strength, break off and have a cup of tea."[9] In this way, the mask will gradually start to break of its own accord as it ceases to be an unconscious means of avoiding reality, and as we become aware of its existence and its purpose, as well as of our own abilities and limitations.

A Prayer of Hope on the Edge of the Abyss[10]

Do not abandon me, O Lord; O my God, do not desert me.
Be attentive to help me, O Lord of my salvation!

---

9   Sophrony, in a 1992 conversation in Essex with Archimandrite Ephraim of Vatopedi, recalling a conversation he had c. 1930. This was the saying that caused him to begin his relationship with St. Silouan. Available online: https://pemptousia.com/2015/07/a-conversation-with-the-elder-sophrony/.

10   Ps. 37:22–23 (38:21–22).

CHAPTER 8

Removing Our Masks

You who rest in the gardens,
The companions turn attentively to your voice;
Let me hear it.

—Song of Songs 8:13

I ENDED THE PREVIOUS CHAPTER on the edge of the abyss, with my masks the only means of psychological survival in the face of total existential despair. What calls me from the abyss is the voice of the Bridegroom, who is Christ. In his homilies on the Song of Songs, St. Gregory of Nyssa says that the wound caused by tearing away my old fleshly humanity (ripping away my masks) is a wound of love, the point of entry for Christ: "O sweet and happy wound, by which life slips through to the inward parts."[1] That is, to remove the masks is to suffer, but unlike the suffering I have endured behind my masks, this suffering is meaningful and creative. Through it I can find the way, truth, and life (John 14:6). If I can begin to remove my masks, then

---

1   Norris, *Gregory of Nyssa*, Homilies 4 and 11, 141 and 347.

perhaps I can begin to see the abyss as the chaos out of which creation is possible, as the nothingness out of which God creates everything.

Behind my masks, I have lived with a chaos of desires. Whenever I have followed my desires, I have never been fulfilled but always led back to the abyss, to nothingness. Faced with the abyss, I have always at this point turned away from reality and retreated back behind the safety of my masks. But deeper and more real than all this, my need for real encounter remains. That need is also the desire to hear the voice of the other calling to me and to respond in truth. To be seen as I truly am, to be heard singing the song of my heart. I am hidden away, and I want to be found. In order to be found, I need others. I must connect. I cannot do this on my own.

So instead of using my imagination to create fantasy—fantastic visions of unreality—I can use it to truly meet the whole different reality of another real person. I can use it to bring me out from the prison behind my mask and connect with another in truth. As C. S. Lewis describes it:

> The true exercise of imagination, in my view, is (a) To help us to understand other people (b) To respond to, and, some of us, to produce, art. But it has also a bad use: to provide for us, in shadowy form, a substitute for virtues, successes, distinctions etc. which ought to be sought outside in the real world . . . After all, almost the main work of life is to come out of our selves, out of the little, dark prison we are all born in.[2]

I can use my imaginative faculty to build and develop an empathy in truth—re-presenting the unique different reality of another within me, rather than using it to avoid understanding and empathizing even with myself by detaching myself from my own reality.

---

2   Letter to Keith Masson, June 3, 1956. *Collected Letters*, 758–759.

Instead of losing the real me in the labyrinth of myself, locking the real me behind the mask, I can begin to step out of myself and into the other, to form real connections that go beyond the physical. This is by definition a process of *ecstasy* (*ek-stasis*—moving out from my own place). My aim is not to achieve some kind of ecstatic feeling (as in my addictive behaviors or fantasies) but to step out from behind my mask of protection to truly connect with the unknown and ultimately unknowable, which will be a transformative experience. In truth, this is the only way to know God at all, as to know Him only rationally is, by definition, impossible. The only way to know God is personally: to meet Him in His uncreated energies and in His creation. And because each human being, made in the image of God, is a microcosm of God, this is true also for any real and meaningful relationship with another human being. We can only truly know anyone personally and interpersonally through encountering them: who they are, how they live out their being, how they relate, and what they create. We can never know another person objectively; this is just a euphemistic cover for objectification.

And encounter is impossible in pornography. Any involvement with pornography means I not only collaborate with the exploitation of people who have been and are being abused and tricked, but I also collude in objectifying them, seeing them merely as objects to use rather than as real human beings to love. I may have little direct control over their experience of their own lives, but I can change the way I see them. I can picture their faces in my mind (or even print an image of a face, if that is possible, to keep in my prayer corner), and I can pray daily for the real person behind the mask:

Save, O Lord, and have mercy on your servant(s) [prostration].
Deliver him/her/them from every tribulation, wrath, and need [prostration],
From every sickness of soul and body [prostration].

Forgive him/her/them every transgression, voluntary and involuntary [prostration].

And do whatever is profitable for our souls [prostration].[3]

Through praying for them, I am transforming my own desires in the light of God's presence. Indeed, the whole process of removing my masks is the process of transforming my desires so that they more closely reflect what they really are in their deepest significance: a desire for union with God. I can lift my masks in the knowledge that my desire for union really can be ultimately fulfilled in perfect union in Christ—in theosis.

Overcoming the addictive pattern is part of this process of removing my masks and transforming my desires. Remember the words of St. Paul: "I do not know what I am accomplishing! . . . I do not do the good I want, but the bad I do not want is what I do in practice! . . . Who will deliver me from this body of death?" (Rom. 7:15–24). I said at the beginning of this section on masks that this is as good a description as any of the addictive process of habitual sin, and this addictive process is the way I maintain my mask: it is what I create to imprison myself in safety.

In the modern world we have seen a lot of research on addiction and ways to help people address it, and while there are many disagreements as to the nature of addiction and therefore what approaches help best, we can learn many useful things from some of the research. Back in the 1970s, a series of experiments on animals tested the addictive nature and effects of drugs such as cocaine and heroin. In one series of particularly influential studies,[4] researchers provided a rat in a cage with an addictive drug on tap and watched to

---

3 Adapted from a prayer "if you wish to pray more diligently for someone" in the *Old Orthodox Prayer Book*, 59.

4 Hari, *Chasing the Scream*, 203–208. These experiments were used as the basis for an anti-drugs television advertisement in the USA in the 1980s.

see how he used it. The rat tried it, began to use it regularly, and then increased his consumption; what followed was a period of bingeing on the drug with small periods of abstinence in between. In the end, he took a lethal overdose. This study has often been quoted as a paradigm of the process of addiction, and it is clear that in some ways I am like that rat: I may try a drug or an experience, I may become addicted to the pleasure but recognize the dangers so that I alternately binge and abstain, and as my life focuses more and more on pursuing these shadow-desires, I may finally end up dead either by misadventure or suicide.

As awareness of these problems grew, at the same time these experiments were going on there was also a rapid growth in twelve-step programs for drug users. These twelve-step programs had started back in the 1950s based on the model of Alcoholics Anonymous (AA, which itself had started in the 1930s). But from the 1970s on, public awareness of addiction began to increase dramatically, and so did various models of assistance, support groups, and therapies that aimed to deal with addiction. These programs developed a lot of the now-standard approaches to addiction, including:

- acknowledging the problem
- admitting that we need help and seeking it out
- examining ourselves and confessing our failings
- finding the desire to change
- making amends
- helping others
- having an accountability partner—a friend we can turn to in moments of weakness
- establishing positive patterns of behavior and practicing them
- replacing our negative, descending life spirals with positive alternatives.

All of these are useful approaches for anyone struggling with an addiction to pornography, just as they are for those addicted to drugs or alcohol. But on their own, they are unlikely to be enough:[5] we need to go deeper. And alongside these approaches, there are other, less helpful voices. For example, we may often hear that more opportunities for actual sexual relationships or experiences would cause the desire for pornography to be subsumed. But this is simply not the case, as many can attest. Relationships do not in themselves protect against pornography use. Of course, we are not likely to hear this advice within the Church, but we might hear a variation of it: "You need to get married." This is a misunderstanding of St. Paul's advice, "If they cannot control themselves, let them marry" (1 Cor. 7:9). Getting married will not magically make these other problems go away or magically provide self-control, and once you are married, it is not acceptable to burn with lust just because it is lust directed at your spouse. No. Marriage opens a path where it is possible for these misdirected desires to be transformed and directed to a fuller union that is more than merely psycho-physical—to a face-to-face union. This kind of union, in the right circumstances, may help us to lift the masks. However, the challenges will still be there, and the ascetic struggle will still be necessary. Getting married is not enough on its own, because it only introduces a context for moving beyond the mask; it does not in itself actualize the removal. But this example of marriage helps us begin to see what is most important. It helps us see how to address the deeper issue, to do more than just

---

5   Even AA's own figures showing that 36 percent of AA participants remain sober long-term (AA 2014 Membership Survey) relate only to those who stay in the program, which may be only about 60 percent, according to Scott O. Lilienfeld and Hal Arkowitz, "Facts and Fictions in Mental Health: Does Alcoholics Anonymous Work?" in *Scientific American MIND* 22, no. 1 (March 2011): 64–65. This study also shows that recovery significantly improves among those who also see a therapist alongside participation in AA.

avoid temptation or even replace a bad habit with a better one. The deeper issue can only be addressed through relationship characterized by creative, life-giving, mutually self-sacrificial love.

Relating in this way means meeting Christ and voluntarily accepting my cross, which I carry as a result both of my own sin and of the sins of others against me. I cannot remove my masks by focusing on fighting a battle against pornography, or against addiction, or against any sin. I can only do it by learning to accept and venerate my cross. This is not easy. I remember some years ago sitting on the floor listening to a sermon during Lent, on the Sunday of the Veneration of the Cross, and hearing about the need to carry one's cross.[6] But then I heard that I need not only to carry my cross, but to venerate it. I thought, *This is way too hard for me. Fine, this Orthodoxy thing is very beautiful, but I think I'll just go home now; I can't do this.* I had understood the need to venerate Christ's Cross but had not appreciated that Christ's Cross and my cross are one—that the cross I carry is continuous with His. It is a shocking thought: that this heavy burden, this weight that I often feel I cannot manage and long to be rid of, is not only something I have to carry, not only something I should somehow be thankful for, but something I should bow down before and kiss. Yet until I learn to venerate the cross I carry, I cannot remove my masks.

The Cross is one of our primary icons—one of the key ways we can look beyond the mask of the fallen world and see God at work. (See color photo insert B.) It is "the weapon of peace, the trophy invincible."[7] It is "the abyss of wonders, the center of desires, the school of virtues, the house of wisdom, the throne of love, the theatre of joys, and the place of sorrows; it is the root of happiness, and the gate of

---

6   Sermon by Fr. Patrick Tishel at Holy Resurrection Orthodox Church, Allston, MA, c. 2010.

7   Kontakion for the Exaltation of the Precious and Life-Giving Cross. *Prayer Book for Orthodox Christians*, 152.

heaven."[8] This is the cross I venerate and the cross I carry. The cross was, in origin, a hated symbol of death, and in fact this is sometimes how I feel about the cross I carry. But in Christ the cross became the symbol of life and self-sacrificial love, the means by which we are freed from sin and by which death is overcome. And my own cross, united to Christ's, can become part of that same process, if I learn to venerate it. Our sin and all that ties it to our masks was set aside when it was nailed to the Cross (Col. 2:14; 2 Cor. 5:21), and as all masks fall away in the power of the Cross, we see the source of all Life and Truth behind them. We need to venerate because it is the only way to see the truth that lies behind the sin. Any sin is a mask of shadows and results in more shiny layers being painted on top to cover the darkness. But with the eyes to see, these masks become veils that can allow us to see something of eternal reality and eternal significance behind them. Only through veneration can we truly understand our masks, and only then can they become icons of resurrection rather than of death, through transformation into glory.

To venerate requires me to face the fear and let go of the attachment to pleasure, which I mentioned above as two key elements of addiction. I face the fear of the abyss that appears to lie on the other side of my mask, and I face the loss of pleasure that sustains my mask and is my counterfeit for the fullness of life I have despaired of ever reaching. Venerating the Cross is where I learn how fear and attachment to pleasure can be transcended and thereby transformed into love and true joy.

My fear is occasionally straight-out terror or panic, but usually it manifests as tension or anxiety. These feelings bubble below the surface, and because I don't know how to face them, they subtly and subconsciously infect all my actions and relationships. This creeping dread, this anxiety, this tension wants to be released, and so I find

---

8   Century I:58 in Traherne, *Centuries of Meditations,* 39.

some way of releasing it without facing it. This is the shadow layer of my mask. I can release it by reducing my inhibitions and awareness through alcohol or drugs, or I can find physical release of tension through sexual behavior, alone or with others. But even if I do this with others, it is not the same as true encounter or relationship.

Deep inside, my fear can build up so that I am afraid to face myself, afraid of the true nature of my being. We often refer to this as self-hatred or self-loathing. Common responses to fear are fight, flight, freeze, or flop (become passive). I might do any of these things, but in the case of self-hatred, this is a fight response turned inward: anger or violence against myself (sometimes combined with a passive or passive-aggressive response to others). If I turn the anger and violence outward, it becomes one of the sources of the desire for the kind of violent pornography that is increasingly prevalent on the internet. This kind of passion is a monstrous hybrid of the fighting passions of anger and violence tied up together with the desiring passions of lust and neediness.

Most of the time, violent anger tied to fear is a veil over a deeper need to grieve. It is my way of fighting back against the loss or absence of something I really need, such as real intimacy. It is my way of refusing to acknowledge or accept that need. Saint John of the Ladder hints at this when he says that an antidote to anger is tears, and that although anger is better expressed (though not directly or aggressively against another) than internalized, the best way to express it is as grief.[9] This applies also to my deep fear, anxiety, or tension: it is a veil covering some loss or lack that I need to grieve rather than hide. So overcoming fear means learning to grieve, which implies learning to share myself, knowing myself, and learning to truly confess.

---

9   Climacus, *Ladder*, 8, 81–84. Tears will quench the flame of anger (8:1). Holding the anger within can build resentment and is "sullying the whiteness of the Dove with black gall" (8:15). Anger is bad, aggressive words are worse, and coming to blows is "utterly inimical" to life in Christ (8:19).

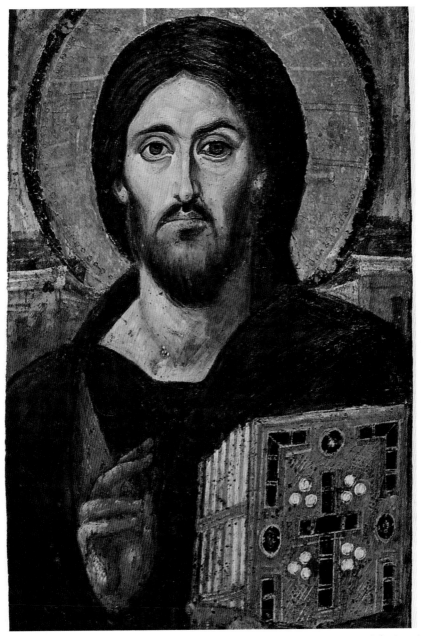

(A) Icon of Christ of Sinai. "I venerate the image of Christ, as God incarnate" (John of Damascus, *Treatise*, I:21).

Christ Pantocrator from Saint Catherine Monastery, Wikimedia Commons.

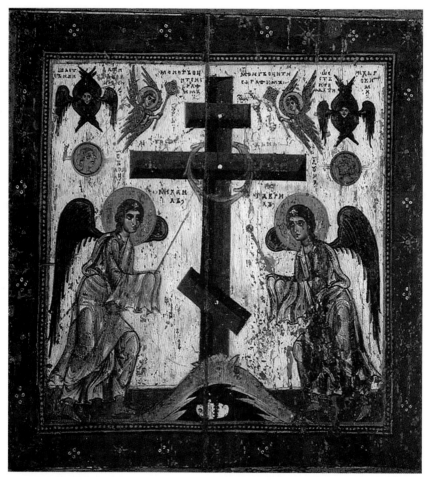

(B) Icon of the Elevation of the Cross. "Thy Cross, O Lord all-merciful, is honored by the whole world, for Thou hast made the instrument of death into a source of life. Sanctify those who venerate it, O God of our fathers, who alone art blessed and greatly glorified" (Matins Canon on the Sunday of the Cross, *Triodion*, 343).

Elevation of the Holy Cross, Alamy Stock Photo.

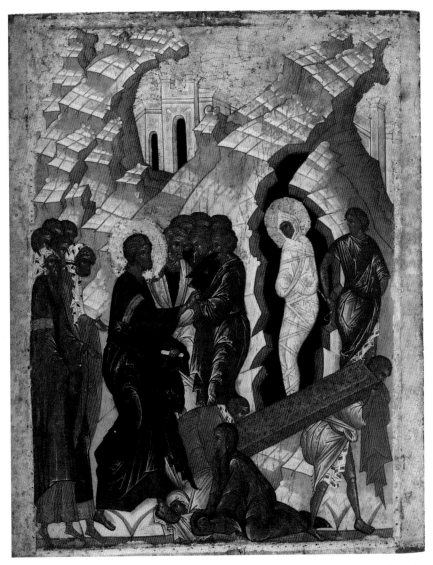

(C) Icon of the Raising of Lazarus. "Since Thou art the Life of the dead, in Thy love for mankind Thou hast turned their sorrow into joy" (Second Canon at Matins on the Saturday of Lazarus, *Triodion*, 480).

The Raising of Lazarus. The Russian Museum, St. Petersburg, Russia, Wikimedia Commons.

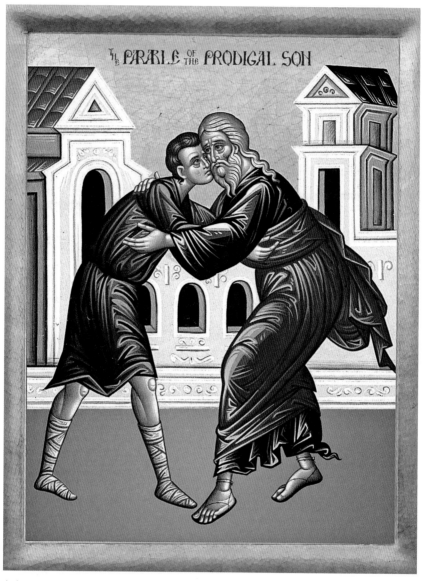

(D) Icon of the Prodigal Son's Return. "Open Thy fatherly embrace now and accept me also as the Prodigal Son, O most merciful Lord, that I may glorify Thee with thanksgiving" (Matins Canon on the Sunday of the Prodigal, *Triodion*, 115).

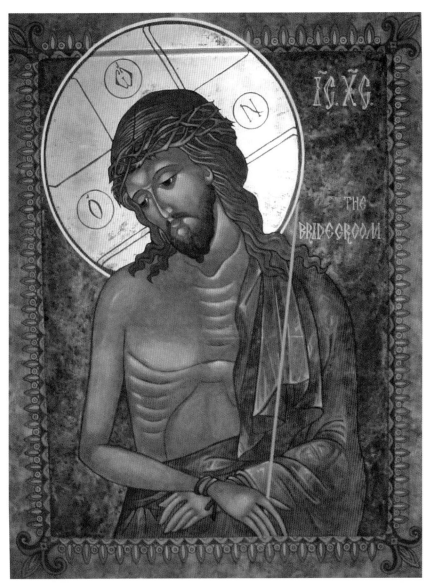

(E) Icon of Christ the Bridegroom. "O Bridegroom, surpassing all in beauty, Thou hast called us to the spiritual feast of Thy bridal chamber. Strip from me the disfigurement of sin, through participation in Thy sufferings; clothe me in the glorious robe of Thy beauty, and in Thy compassion make me feast with joy at Thy Kingdom" (Aposticha at Matins on Holy Tuesday, *Triodion*, 528).

Icon of Christ the Bridegroom, Wikimedia Commons.

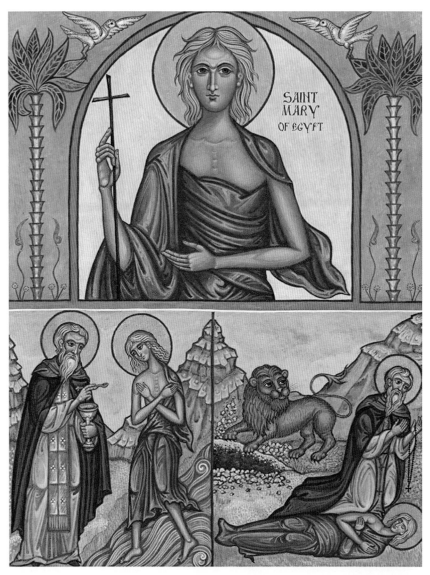

(F) Icon of St. Mary of Egypt. "With the streams of thy tears thou hast watered all the wilderness, and caused the fruits of repentance to spring up for us: therefore, O saint, we celebrate thy memory" (Saturday Vespers for the Sunday of St. Mary of Egypt, *Triodion*, 449).

"Truly God did not lie when He promised that when we purify ourselves we shall be like Him. Glory to Thee, Christ our God!" (The words St. Zosimas spoke when he brought Communion to St. Mary of Egypt. "The Life of Our Holy Mother Mary of Egypt," *Great Canon*, 93.)

Icon of St. Mary of Egypt with scenes from her life. Copyright © Uncut Mountain Supply, Manton, MI, used by permission. All rights reserved.

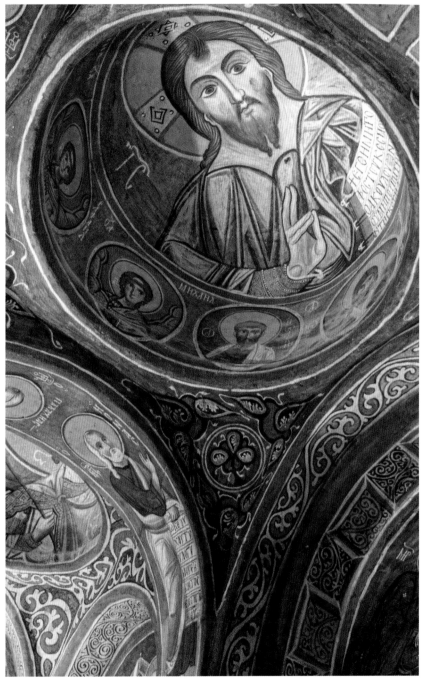

(G) Icon of Christ Pantokrator. "The one who sees Me has seen the Father" (John 14:9).

Pantocrator in Dome, Shutterstock © Matyas Rehak.

Of course, rather than grieving, sharing, and confessing, I would prefer to avoid suffering and seek a feel-good escapism in my addiction. I would rather avoid the Reality of what lies behind the veil of creation and see pornographically instead of iconologically. But if I indulge my escapism, I will never be able to remove my masks and enjoy the true depths of intimacy and communion that in my escapism I desire to meet but can in fact only imagine.

This feel-good escapism works on physical, psychological, and spiritual levels simultaneously. On the physical level, it manifests in brain chemicals such as dopamine, noradrenaline, oxytocin, and serotonin—the drugs we all prescribe and manufacture for ourselves in our own bodies in response to our thoughts, fantasies, and behaviors. If we keep returning to our habitual soothing behaviors, we become more dependent on these neurochemicals, which in turn gradually change the makeup of our brains.[10]

On a psychological level we describe escapism in terms of established patterns of behavior, reactions to past hurt and broken relationships, patterns of avoiding life's difficulties, and not succeeding in living up to our ideals (doing the evil we do not want to do). If we face difficult thoughts and memories, the temptation to avoid them by escaping into something pleasurable can be hard to resist. This can even be such a subconscious process that we may find ourselves in our soothing behaviors before even being consciously aware of what we are trying to avoid.

On the spiritual level, we experience escapism as degrees of separation from God (that is, from the Reality found behind all masks and veils). So if we avoid the difficult reality of a situation and move into our soothing avoidance behaviors, we move further from the realm

---

10   See for example Maté, *Realm of Hungry Ghosts*, 173–180; Doidge, *Brain That Changes*, 124–139.

of the iconic veils—facilitating the connection to God and ultimate Reality—and further into the realm of masks.

Removing my masks effectively, then, needs to be done in a way that involves all these levels of my being. Of course, in reality, these levels are not separable from each other: the body, mind, and spirit all affect each other. In the negative spiral of the masks, body, mind, and spirit combine into a phronema that darkens my vision, paints more layers onto my own masks, and constantly decreases my ability to see anything beyond the masks of others. This is the phronema of the masks or of the flesh.

We have seen above that change is possible in the spiritual, psychological, and emotional realms. When we look at the physical level more closely, we see that here, too, change is possible. The concept of neuroplasticity—the word for the constant reworking of the brain's pathways—demonstrates how this works.[11] Much recent research has shown how our brains change themselves in response to our experiences, our environment, our thoughts and actions. This acknowledges on the physical level that we are constantly a work in progress, that God's creation is not over, and that we are partaking in it—including in the ongoing creation of ourselves. It shows that no mask is permanent: we always have the option of change on every level of our being, no matter how deeply rooted our past difficulties and our present avoidant or escapist coping strategies.

I have already quoted St. Isaac the Syrian above: "This life has been given to you for repentance; do not waste it in vain pursuits." There is no pursuit more vain than my soothing, escapist behaviors. Whether I like it or not, they are by nature targeted only at the surface of my life, at making things appear better for a time. And as we have seen, as I practice them, rather than making a real positive change, I make it harder and harder for that real positive change—the removal of my

---

11   See, Doidge, for example.

masks—to happen. Instead of continuing to follow these vain pursuits, I need to redesign my life into a habitual pattern of repentance, because whatever I practice will continually form the person I am becoming, body, mind, and spirit.

Conversely, if I practice those vain pursuits, I am still co-creating myself, but I am creating myself not via the narrow path of repentance, which moves toward fulfilling my deepest desires in union with God, but on the broad and easy path of separation from God and toward the prison of being enslaved in my own desires while never being able to fulfill them. Yes, the work is urgent, because every delay forms me just a little bit more in the wrong way, away from the person I really want to be—the person God created me to be. Every delay reinforces the masks, and my deeper desire (if I could but see it clearly) is to remove them.

As I indulge my addiction, I form myself more and more into that pattern of fear, of running after the feel-good pleasure, of avoidance of the path toward fulfillment. On the physical level, I achieve this either with or without chemicals that I put into my body. Doctors advise nicotine patches for those trying to give up smoking, but they help in fewer than 20 percent of cases because, as with any addiction, the chemicals coming from outside the body are only a small part of the story.[12] It is not so much what I put into my body that makes me impure as what I already have inside there. I generate my own chemicals (neurotransmitters) to imprison myself further in the cage of fear and misdirected desire behind the masks. This is why it is reasonable to describe a behavior like pornography use as an addiction in the same way as the compulsion to use drugs or alcohol is an addiction.

But of course, as we have seen above, addiction is not all about the physical level—the psychological, spiritual, and relational levels are significant, too. The rat in the cage kept returning to his drug

---

12   See Hari, *Chasing the Scream,* 221.

until he killed himself by overdose. This demonstrates the physical effect neatly. But some scientists in the 1970s and '80s saw something missing in that experiment, so they came up with another experiment to test their hypothesis—popularly known as the Rat Park experiment.[13]

The scientists thought perhaps the rat lacked something in his life. He had nothing else to do, after all, so why not turn to drugs? So they designed a sort of rat's paradise instead of the original cage. This paradise included lots of activities and other rats to socialize with. It was a different world. And the results were different, too. Those rats tried the drug, but they didn't become addicted, and they didn't overdose. Instead, they had ways to add meaning to their lives. In fact, when the researchers moved rats who were already addicted to the drug from the lonely cages to the paradise, these addicted rats would overcome their addiction, even though the drug was still on offer. With addiction, nothing is as simple as it looks: there is always something behind the masks, and there is always an interaction between the physical, psychological, spiritual, and relational.

So this is another important lesson in developing a life resilient to addictions. As with Rat Park, changing my environment (in the broadest sense) will make a difference. Developing new patterns, filling my life with constructive pursuits rather than vain ones, and—especially—developing meaningful relationships will help me to begin to lift my masks. Throwing the demons out of the house of my soul will only leave room for more demons to squat and hold demonic parties (Matt. 12:43–45). I need to fill the house with guests who have my better interests at heart, those who bring me real fulfillment, that is also real joy, and enable me to show my deeper, truer self.

Of course, we do not live in a park all the time, and it is well-known that when times are hard, we find it difficult to be the best

---

13   There is a summary of these experiments in Hari, 207–208.

version of ourselves. This is one reason we practice in anticipation of the hard times to come. Through ascetic efforts such as fasting, we explore whether we can make life more difficult and yet live well. Can we forgo food and still not give way to anger or lust? Can we face hard times and keep free of addiction? Our ascetic practice is one of the ways we clean the demons out of our souls. The danger is that through cleansing we may unintentionally provide an inviting open house for more demons. This is where the practice of *nepsis* comes in, which means the sober wakefulness or watchfulness that guards the soul, especially after a time of cleansing. Saint Hesychios the Priest defines *nepsis* as "a continual fixing and halting of thought at the entrance to the heart."[14] The word came into Christian usage through the letter of St. Peter: "Be sober and watchful *[νήψατε]*; wake up! Your accuser the devil like a roaring lion is walking around seeking whom to devour" (1 Pet. 5:8). This is why our ascetic practice is always combined with a sober attentiveness in the eye of our hearts to the presence of God.

This combination of ascetic practice with nepsis is vital because I do need to master, comprehend, and assimilate my biological and physical desires so that they do not make my masks so densely layered that I cannot see through to the spiritual reality beyond. Here I am, stuck in the outermost layer, the physical, as if I look at the icon and all I can see is some paint and wood. It is as if the center and goal of life is the flesh—that body of death. Instead, death has been trampled down by death so that we can be invited into a greater and fuller and more real life.

And yet, however much I practice and struggle, I will keep falling back into that masked life. If the great ascetics failed, I will also fail. Failure is not only an option, it is inevitable—but even failure can work for good. The Cross teaches us this: the point at which it seems

---

14 "On Watchfulness and Holiness," in *Philokalia* Vol. 1, 163.

I have met my worst failure, the lowest point, the end of all hopes can actually be the beginning of a fullness of life I cannot even imagine.

Once the Crucifixion had become inevitable, in the shadow of the Cross, most of the disciples and apostles did not even last long enough to hear "My God, My God, why have You forsaken Me?" (Matt. 27:46) before they dispersed and fled, their hopes in tatters. And yet, had they but understood, they were standing on the verge of victory over death. Death is always part of this life, but it has lost its power to destroy. So when I fail, I can accept this as the normal way, and, looking to the Cross, I can pick myself up and go on living my life. This is true in the big things and the small, both in the crises and in the ascetic practice by which we strengthen ourselves to be ready for them. Saint Gregory of Sinai advises us thus: "If you eat too much, repent and try again. Always act like this—lapsing and recovering again . . . and you will be at peace, wisely converting such lapses into victories, as Scripture says."[15]

Each failure is in itself also the opportunity for greater self-knowledge and awareness, if I am attentive. The more I learn to see beyond the mask and perceive what I am actually lacking, the more I am likely to be able to grieve my lack and move my life toward true fulfillment, rather than continually emptying the house of demons only to allow new ones in. I may be able to learn some of the triggers that prompt my run into escapism—feelings, moods, particular encounters, relationships, or situations that cause me to hold tightly to my masks. And when I look at the picture on my mask, I may begin to understand what I get from the escapism, what my mode of escape symbolizes about my deeper need.

When I can accept my failures, I may also begin to learn humility, which I cannot do without accepting myself as I truly am, including all my weaknesses. In fact, as I learn to venerate my cross, I also learn

---

15   "On Prayer: Seven Texts," in *Philokalia* Vol. 4, 281.

to be thankful for the failures and losses that teach me the path of humility. These failures and losses are also blessings. They teach me that humility is not found in ignoring my own needs and pushing myself beyond my ability to cope. To do that actually demonstrates narcissistic arrogance. Humility means acknowledging my own needs and my inability to cope, and asking for the necessary help and support. This may involve finding a way to meet my needs directly, or it may involve acknowledging the need, exploring why it can't be met directly, and reflecting on what it reveals about my deeper needs and the path to ultimately finding fulfillment for these.

In the meantime, I can set up for myself an orderly and liturgical life that builds in supporting structures and ascetic practice. Building a liturgical life is not only about regular participation in the Liturgy and the sacramental life of the Church—though this is central—but it is about all of life. As well as committing to regular confession and participation in the Liturgy and other services, I can follow the fasts of the Church and incorporate into them fasting from social and other modern media. I can structure my days to involve a regular return to the present moment, as that is the only real time in which I can truly live (since the future is an imaginary mask and the past is a fixed image). I can do this by regular practice of the Jesus Prayer; by observing regular prayer times throughout the day using the *Book of Hours* (*Horologion*), the rule of St. Pachomius, or another prayer rule recommended by my spiritual father; and by using the prayers before and after meals and the prayers before tasks and events that are commonly found in Orthodox prayer books. One way or another, it is possible with practice to build in prayers throughout any kind of day: if circumstances permit nothing else, internal prayer from memory, repetition of the Jesus Prayer, and cultivating the prayer of the heart is possible. As well as regular contact with other people (supportive and encouraging people in particular), building in moments of intentional interaction with the rest of the created world can also help—walking in nature, or even engaging in simple, intentional physical contact—connecting my physical senses with the created world.

Our home is a little church, and creating the right sort of context and atmosphere is of great importance here, too. To do this, we can pay attention to things such as the focal point of our home—what our eyes are drawn toward, and how we set up, maintain, and use our icon corner. We can also notice how our home is decorated in general, what the activity of our home life circles around, and how our days at home begin and end.

The liturgical life is a life of veils, but never of masks. In the liturgical life, our physical bodies are fully engaged, but rather than being locked in masks that obscure the life beyond, all our physical actions are veils that constantly direct us to the fuller life of the spirit beyond the flesh. In order to participate in the liturgical life in the most meaningful way, I have to participate in all humility as my true self. From behind a mask, as we have seen, true communion is impossible. Allowing Christ to lift off the mask I have made for myself is precisely what makes me worthy to participate in Communion—to receive His Body and Blood for eternal life. Masks are some of the earthly cares the Cherubic Hymn calls me to lay aside, and I have to present myself just as I really am.

Learning to lift the mask liturgically in church and in prayer is the beginning. I can go on to integrate the rest of my experience into the same pattern. When I start to feel the desire to satisfy myself in one of my habitual sins—which is a mask over my true needs—can I, rather than rushing to satisfy the immediate lustful desire, sit with it to find out what kind of discomfort or pain I feel when I refuse to indulge the desire? Recognizing the desire as an image on a mask, can I refuse to be drawn in and instead look behind it and discern a deeper meaning: where it is trying to send me and why; how I might truly find fulfillment rather than repeatedly diving into a moment of false ecstasy that dies into nothingness?

If I have begun to see beyond the masks, I can sit in this desire without the possibility of immediate fulfillment because I have started to live in reality. The fantasy seemed preferable because that way, at least I got a taste of what I wanted. This way is so much harder—just desolation. I am left unconnected, existentially alone. This is not a loss I am usually willing to bear. What can make me willing to bear it? What enables me to bear it? My whole body cries out for connection, and this is the icon of my soul's deeper cry. I may be angry that connection is not available to me. I may be empty and desolate with a sadness beyond tears—a sadness that I cannot do this. I cannot make this connection that my whole self seems to have been made for, to cry out for. It seems to make sense that if I cannot look so deeply into the eyes of another soul and have them look so deeply into mine in reality, then why can I not at least have the fantasy of this moment?[16] How can the everyday reality of attempted relationship, with its petty issues, imperfect physical experiences, and misunderstandings, ever help me reach this intense and perfect experience that I desire?

It can help because I need not only to see and to feel, but actually to be seen and to be felt in reality—in a true encounter, face to face. Connection is at the heart of this desire, and ultimately, I need the connection to be real. The fantasy connection, wherein I am seen only in fantasy and touched only in fantasy, is not enough. Even with a real person, when they see me physically it is not enough. Though I need to be seen in my physical body, I need that seeing to be more than pornographic—I need it to be iconographic. I need the other to

---

16 In the Tolstoy short story, "Happy Ever After," Masha, on realizing that the earlier intensity of love with her husband has passed away, is tempted to hold onto the memory of it rather than accepting her current reality. Tolstoy, 97–98.

look at my body and see through it to the soul beyond. I would also like it to be iconological—for the other to see my body and venerate it not so much for what it is physically as for the meaning it reveals: who I truly am in all my fullness. That is the only thing that will ultimately fulfill this desire. That is also therefore what I can aim to offer to others.

I cannot get there without living through and into the reality of my weakness. In order to do this, I must listen to my body and to my emotional responses—not in order to react out of them, but to be aware of what they are, aware of what I am saying to myself. My senses and emotions are rational responses to my experience and my life, and I need not run from them into some self-soothing mechanical response. Rather, I can see them as a dial or measure indicating something about my life, about my experience, about myself. Instead of running to soothing, can I note down or journal what I am feeling and what immediately preceded it? Then I can lay those thoughts aside as the earthly cares they are and move to a favorite icon to gaze on the face there, without need for words. Having thus begun to connect with the reality of myself through bringing myself into relation with God through His saints, I can at some future point return to my note or my journal to see what clarity I may have acquired. If I still do not understand, I can take it back to the icon and pray; I can take it as part of my self-examination to confession.

Thus I begin to engage this process of ascetic practice in the context of prayer and an ordered liturgical life. I seek humble honesty within myself and in encounters with others. I learn to overcome fear and voluntarily accept and sit within my real sense of suffering and loss. I practice venerating the Cross and my own cross. And through all this, I begin to learn how to remove my masks, and in doing so both come to know and begin to reveal my true self.

A Prayer of Life[17]

We venerate Thy Cross, O Master, and we glorify Thy holy Resurrection.

---

17 Sung at the veneration of the Cross on the Sunday of the Cross in Great Lent. *Triodion*, 348.

PART 3

Veils

Since the creation of the world His invisible things, His eternal power and deity, have been clearly perceived in created things.

—Romans 1:20

CHAPTER 9

Veils and What They Reveal

A T THE END OF THE previous section, I said that our liturgical life is a life of veils. In the Liturgy, everything is not just what it appears to be at first glance—everything works on multiple levels. Each action and each interaction functions as a veil—it covers what is invisible with what is visible in order to reveal it. Like an icon, it connects the facts of this created world to the deeper truths of the spiritual world. Unlike masks, veils allow two-way communication and two-way visibility. And when we leave the church, we continue to see God through His creation. In this sense, the whole psycho-physical world is a veil over the deeper, eternal reality. Similarly, we can see the outline of the soul of a person through the veil of their physical and behavioral being, and we can see that the person, being made in the image of God, also reveals God to us.

We have already seen that this veil can be darkened, hardened, painted, layered, and formed into a mask to obscure what lies beneath. The contrast between veil and mask is that the veil, like an icon, communicates the presence of the person, whereas the mask obscures and gradually destroys that presence. Iconography is a Mystery of the Church (it is sacramental) because it both embodies a personal presence and introduces us into that presence (according to the proclamations of the Seventh Ecumenical Council),[1] and this is the nature of veils. In contrast to masks, which cover in order to conceal, veils, through covering, reveal. In this life, things of ultimate significance are veiled, and yet the veils make visible the contours of eternity.

Veils are another way to speak of the simultaneously *now* and *not yet* nature of this life, in which everything we experience in our present moment has an eternal significance that is yet to be fully revealed. But we can already begin to perceive everything of eternal significance through the veils—even God Himself, as St. Paul says (Rom. 1:20).

When we perceive beyond the veil, we gain an understanding deeper than the simple image of the created form as it appears to our eyes and brain. As we saw in previous chapters, our imagination is our image-making faculty. We do not have it in order to conjure up things that are disconnected from reality; rather, it is given to us as an organ of seeing. It exists to present images that are true—images that, like icons, participate in ultimate truth. In this the imagination can function as a noetic vision, in contrast to our physical vision, which, like the language we use to describe it, is tied to our physical senses.

Language is itself a veil—it always stands between us and the reality we are trying to communicate or trying to perceive. C. S. Lewis, in one of his talks,[2] discussed some people's objection to the kind of "religious language" we use, such as when we say things like "He came down from heaven," as if heaven were "up there." But it is a clear image (in our imagination, we see it), and it communicates something that is true—that there is a sense in which the Incarnation was a descent, not in physical or topological terms, but in terms

1   "[B]y the representation of the icon . . . we remember all the prototypes and we are introduced into their presence." Evdokimov, *Art of the Icon*, 178.

2   A talk titled "Is Theology Poetry?" given November 6, 1944, to the Oxford Socratic Club and published in *The Weight of Glory*.

of being a self-emptying. Those who object to this language might prefer to say something they think of as less metaphorical, something like "God entered space-time." But, as C. S. Lewis points out, those words only substitute a different movement ("entering") and a different place (called "space-time") for the original "coming down" in a vertical movement from a heaven that is "up there." Either way, the images and language we use function as veils that cover the deeper truth beyond, because we have no way to speak of it directly. Because we are bound to our physical senses and language about them, in this world we cannot see "face to face" but must see "through a glass, darkly." That is, the face we can see is only the surface. My true face communicates so much more about me, but the physical and behavioral alone cannot encompass or express it. So neither ultimately real nor fully literal communication is possible in this world. Despite this, language and images can illuminate the deeper reality behind what we say and see. By covering, the veil reveals.

How exactly does the veil both cover and reveal what lies behind it? Think of an invisible man. You can't see him, obviously; he's invisible. But throw a sheet over him, and his outline becomes visible: you begin to see him. What you now see truly helps you to understand what's there, even though you do not see the fullness. It allows you to imagine what you otherwise could not see but is really there.

Similarly, an icon is not the fullness of reality itself, but it connects us to that fullness. It expresses to us what we cannot otherwise see, even though it is really there. In this sense, an icon is a veil, and this is part of why the icon is the "safeguard of the Orthodox faith"[3]— because it is a constant reminder to us of what we cannot see with our eyes alone.

There is a stark contrast between that veil of the iconic presence and the use of the image in much modern media, where, rather than

---

3   *Triodion*, 300.

revealing the truth of things unseen, the image is carefully cultivated to provoke the senses or the passions, to communicate a specific message, to hide what those who craft it either do not see or do not want us to see. In other words, a literal, physical image is presented as a mask. If I look at pornography, it is the mask I want to see, not the veil. Pornography is about closing the deeper meaning and looking for a static, objectified reality to meet my needs.

In contrast, venerating an icon, I am drawn into life in Christ, which is about opening myself to a dynamic relationship—with the risk that I will be changed but also the possibility of finding true fulfillment. This openness to the other means having the humility to know I cannot create myself under my own power—I am not God and cannot create ex nihilo. I need rather to find myself as I am in Christ, and to do this, I need others. The path is to love God with all my heart, and my neighbor—every icon of Christ around me—as myself. I need to meet God in Christ in the Church and in the world, sacramentally in the Holy Mysteries and iconologically in other people. The path is also about *agnosia* (unknowing) in relationship with the other—like the Theotokos, we ponder these things in our hearts, remain faithful when called upon to act, and maintain courage in the waiting. This unknowing is the empty wooden board we offer to God, who will paint our true face on it.

An icon painter works in the same way, by creating consecutive layers of color on an empty board. Each layer functions as a veil, which, when superimposed over the previous one, partly conceals it, but in doing so begins to reveal the finished icon. This is how creation both covers and yet manifests its Creator.[4] And, just like the icon painter, God starts with nothing, covers it with different physical layers, and *we* come into being—individual, real persons in the image of God, each of us a veil with the potential to make God visible, each of us an

---

4   For more on this, see Manoussakis, *God after Metaphysics*, 32–33.

icon of ultimate Reality. Our role, like that of the icon, is to participate in what we symbolize: to live in the life of God, making that life manifest in the world and seeing it reflected back in the light of the other images of God, the other icons of Christ, the people around us.

The icon, and our ability to see beyond the physical world in general, is the imaginative, creative power of humanity in action. It is the flipside of the power of our fantasy to obscure reality, which moves us into the unreal world of the mask. Thinking back to the invisible man: if, after throwing the sheet over him, we then put a painted mask on top, we cover up what before was our chance to make him out. This makes it harder for us to imagine the truth of the person under the veil. The man behind the mask is now completely unknown. We have no way of knowing whether the mask relates to him at all and no way to truly encounter him. Saint John Climacus tells us that "a lie is the destruction of love,"[5] and St. Nikolaj of Žiča says that "love is the method of comprehension."[6] So while the mask obscures because it lies about reality and makes true love and true knowledge impossible, the veil reveals because it allows both love and understanding to flow and relationship to begin.

My masks are my attempt to save and build my own life, and yet, when I put one on, I lose my life. If I persist in holding onto the mask, at the end of all things, as we have seen, there will be nothing left behind the mask, because the person hiding there in isolation will have shriveled up into nothing. Without God, that nothing behind the mask is just the nothing it was before creation began. And yet, with God, out of nothing comes everything. He creates ex nihilo. In a sense, we can say that through love He imagines everything into being.

In a true relationship, a relationship of love in which we can have true intimacy, we look on the veils that reveal the truth of who is

---

5   Climacus, *Ladder* 12:2, 94.
6   Letter 36, "To a Theologian B," in Velimirovich, *Missionary Letters*, 67.

underneath. We know that the person we look on—every person—is in the image of God, an icon of Christ. We are able to love the reality of that person even in the face of his or her fallenness, because even that fallenness is a veil over the ultimate truth of the perfect human being he or she is to be.

But as I begin to lift my masks that obscure and replace them with veils that reveal, I need to consider how much I should reveal and in what way: there are things I need to reveal and things that it is appropriate to keep covered—like Noah's nakedness (Gen. 9). My spiritual veils are in some ways parallel to my physical clothes. Clothes cover my nakedness without concealing my body's contours—though I can of course use clothes to hide my body or to adorn and display myself in a specific way. Similarly, I can either veil my inner life without concealing myself, or I can use masks to misdirect or hide. What I cannot do with my inner life, the way I can with my body, is to reveal it in a natural nakedness—though in the closest and most honest earthly relationships, I can begin to perceive how, in the fullness of eternal life, this will become possible. In this life, it would not be appropriate to let all my internal processes ooze out of me in every relationship and every encounter with another person, just as it would not be appropriate to go about naked.

There is a time to reveal and a time to keep things behind the veil. Although I need to share and connect, I do not want my internal life and struggles to burden or tempt others, or to be an indulgence which would tempt me to make a new mask for myself. So discernment is required. But this does not mean hiding: I do not want to obscure myself in any relationship. I need to create a veil that preserves my dignity by covering—but a veil, unlike a mask, covers not so much by concealing as by revealing the deeper personal reality beneath. I know that I am not defined by my sins, nor by my temptations, my hurts, and my past: this fallen world is but a shadow of a more glorious ultimate reality. I know that what lies ahead is a union with the one perfect human being—a union so complete and a light so bright that when it shines on all these sins and hurts, even they will be seen ultimately to be glorious, just as the wounds on His hands and feet are glorious.

I can begin to perceive these glories through the veil because, in contrast to the mask with its painted counterfeit of a face, "the icon depicts nothing, it reveals."[7] The infinite regression of the veils of creation always illuminates, whereas the mask obscures. Veils invite, masks mislead; veils suggest, masks impose; veils offer, masks enforce; veils can be penetrated, masks shield against any piercing; veils invite, masks repel; veils are vulnerable, masks are invulnerable.

When I stand in front of the icon and pray, it is my opportunity to be seen through the veil, holding nothing back. If I hold something back, if I am not willing to be fully seen, I begin to turn my veils into masks. If I do not hold anything back, then to confess in front of the icon of Christ or His Mother is to open myself in full vulnerability, to allow all my desires into my awareness, and to hold them up in my mind's eye in the light of the image of Christ or the Theotokos. And I know that in the face of all this, the holy presence mediated by the icon and the reality of the love that flows from the icon to me is unchanged by whatever I may bring. I need have no fear, and I need hold nothing back. In love and trust, I can open everything in and of myself, no matter how disordered, how confused, how damaged and messed up by my life, my own actions, and the actions of others.

To stand in front of the icon and pray in this way is to voluntarily enter a sacred space, a liminal space of both mediated presence and continued absence. The veil in its revelation gives us a taste of the fullness, but the fullness is still not *now*. How do I respond? Do I want

---

7   "Икона ничего не изображает, она являет": the iconographer Archimandrite Zinon. "Archimandrite Zinon (Theodore)," Our Church of St. Anastasia, accessed July 30, 2022, http://weischeitgmeilcom2011.blogspot .com/2013/01/blog-post_3.html, (my translation).

to stay in this liminal place with all its discomforts? Surely I want to break through to the other side in all its fullness. But in fear that the fullness of light and warmth will be too much for my fragile soul, or exhausted by the discomforts of liminality, I may want to put the mask on and retreat from the battle. No matter how uncomfortable it is behind the mask, it is still better than the unknowing and vulnerability of liminality and the need for courage in the face of what lies on the other side. Can God ultimately accept me and receive me into full union with Him? This seems impossible! Do I really want this, anyway? Or would I prefer a safer, masked ability to control exactly how much I give—and a degree of control at least to limit what I receive?

A Prayer of New Life[8]

O Thou Who by Thy divine power didst raise Lazarus,
Raise also me who am corrupt with passions
and have lain for many years in the tomb of unrepentance,
that raised by Thy voice I may sing as one who is saved: Alleluia!
(See color photo insert C.)

---

8   Akathist to the Resurrection of Christ, Kontakion 3. *Akathists*, 92.

CHAPTER 10

Veneration and Relationship

MY EXPERIENCE VENERATING ICONS VARIES. Sometimes I fail to give it my full attention, when I am self-conscious in front of others who wait behind me or when I am rushing on to the next thing. Or sometimes I feel too much shame, and I don't want to be opened up in front of this window on eternity. But essentially, when I stand in prayer before a holy icon, an icon set apart for veneration, I face an opportunity to connect with the world beyond my physical senses, to glorify God in His Creation, to express my adoration of Him with my whole self—body, mind, and spirit—and to join my whole self to Christ's body, the Church. This is why the veneration of icons is central to our worship, as the well-known iconographer Archimandrite Zinon says:

> The icon is embodied prayer. It is created in prayer and for prayer, which is the driving force of the love of God, the desire for Him as perfect beauty. Therefore, the icon in the true sense cannot exist without the Church. As a form of preaching the Gospel, as a testimony of

the Church to the Incarnation, the icon is an integral part of the service, along with church singing, architecture, ritual.[1]

"To venerate" means "to show reverence to"; it is about submission, about humbling myself, about making myself vulnerable. When I bow, I show vulnerability by looking down and exposing my neck. When I make a prostration, I show even more vulnerability and submission as I put my face to the ground. So when I venerate, I make obeisance before something or someone that is highly valued, respected, and trusted. And kissing, of course, is a sign of relationship, of greeting, and of love. Knowing what veneration of a holy image is, then, what do I make of pornography? A pornographic image is an anti-icon in the sense that if I use pornography, I engage in an act that is a mockery of veneration. The desire that I show for the image of God is here characterized by possession and dominance in an act that abuses the image of God.

However, a pornography user in front of porn reflects some of the veneration of an icon in pale or distorted ways: There is an element of submission, especially for the habitual user or addict whose ability to break free is limited. There is a parody of humility in the exposure and in the opening of one's vulnerability in front of an inanimate object. And there is certainly a degree of value assigned to the porn—even if there is no respect for the reality of the person or persons portrayed there—and an element of lust, which is a parody or mask of love. Hence, we can say that both praying with an icon and using pornography are forms of veneration: one holy, the other blasphemous or idolatrous.

There are different ways of standing in front of an image. We can venerate; we can be indifferent; we can abuse. We can lust; we can destroy. We can love; we can hate. We can show our true face through

---

1   "Archimandrite Zinon."

the veil, or we can hide behind a mask. We can open our spiritual eyes and see through the veils of this world, or we can make every face a mask and see nothing of truth. Every one of these moments is a moment in eternity, a potential transformational encounter, and the effect my own feelings and actions have on me can be as great as the effect of the image itself.[2]

Our experience before the image confirms what the Fathers tell us: that the veneration we give to the icon passes to the prototype. When we venerate an icon, the veneration passes to the saint herself. And yet this in itself does not distinguish a holy icon from any other image. For example, if I kiss the photograph of someone I love, I express my love for the person portrayed in the photograph, not for the photograph itself. It's not that I don't love the image; I do, but I love the image because it is an image of that person.

However, there is a popular use of the word *icon* that is one step removed from how veneration and love pass from image to archetype: when people speak of celebrities as icons. But of what are they icons? Fans will keep pictures of these so-called "icons" and may even treat them with reverence, and in some cases even kiss them. But in some important ways, this process differs from that of the holy icon or the photograph of a loved one. First, these images have often been manipulated: they are professionally made photographs, designed to create a particular impression of the person portrayed—designed, therefore, specifically to prevent relating through the veil. It is unlikely that there can be any real relationship between the one looking at the image and the true reality of the person it portrays. And not only that, but the reason the fan has for what is even popularly called *idolizing* the person portrayed in the image likely has more to do with fantasy than with reality.

---

2   For more on how these moments change us, see chapters 4 and 8 above, including the discussion on neuroplasticity and the way we co-create ourselves.

And when we take a step further, we arrive at pornography proper. A pornographic image is an anti-icon because it prevents relating through veils. It takes all the meaning and significance of the image and perverts it, as evil always takes what is good and twists it. Everything evil, having no reality of its own, is just a perversion of something good. One reason we may find evil alluring is precisely that it still always reflects something of the good character of its origin in the creation that God saw and said was good. Pornography is an anti-icon because it prevents real relationship. And since the link between the image and the archetype is broken, true veneration is impossible. There is no longer any possibility of love or respect passing to the prototype (the person) and through that prototype, to the ultimate archetype, God Himself, who has made that person in His image. And more extreme than this, some pornography is even explicitly demonic; it abuses and exploits the link between image and archetype to deliberately lead the user to connect to the demonic world.

So all these things are images: holy icons, photos of loved ones, published pictures of celebrities, pornographic pictures or videos—but the holy icon defines for us what an image should be. It also teaches us that the appropriate way to approach all images is with attention to the prototype and with respect, love, and gratitude for all that God has created, which reflects something of His life. Even in the case of explicitly idolatrous or demonic images, if I were pure in heart and eye, I would be able to see the misdirection of the demonic mask as a veil in itself and find a way to relate to the angelic life beyond. But in my fallen and weakened state, I have to be realistic about my own abilities, and this means, in proper humility, I need to turn from certain images because of my own sin. There are times when I am not yet able to relate through the veil because I am unable to resist the temptation of the mask's misdirection.

It should be apparent by this point that there is no clear distinction between veils and masks. What looks like a mask to me in my sin will be just a veil to a purified eye, and through that veil, such a person will connect to greater holiness. I, on the other hand, will remain unaware of what truly lies beyond, and I will be caught up in the misdirection of this fallen world. This means that I may look at an image and see a pornographic picture, while another may look at the same image and see a person made in God's image, a person it is possible to love purely, and through that love connect to God's love.

This is why I believe it is necessary to see pornography in the light of iconography. But when I have talked about these topics before, some people have written to me, concerned that it is inappropriate to talk about iconography and pornography in the same discussion. They suppose that to do so—to make any comparison at all between them—degrades the holy icons to the level of pornography. But this is a false division of the human person; there are not two separate kinds of people or two separate kinds of desire. There is only human desire, though through it we can aim either toward wholeness and perfect communion or toward something less than perfect wholeness. Enforcing an unbridgeable divide between pornography and iconography would make diagnosis impossible, because we would be unable to place the illness in the context of its healing. And in fact, it would mean suffering from the same fear and the same despair that makes the temptation to pornography possible in the first place.

To juxtapose iconography and pornography is to cast the light of one onto the darkness of the other. This makes not only the parallels but more particularly the contrast clear—just as in the Incarnation, God came as a perfect human being to walk among imperfect, defiled, and degraded human beings. He was one person among many other people and yet a man shining with the light of perfection, the perfect human being, the perfect image of the Father, in perfect union with Him. A man, but not just another man: God Himself. Hence, it is important to acknowledge that iconography and pornography both involve the creation and use of images, and both commonly present to us images of created men and women. But there is a difference between the light that shines from the one, which illuminates the truth and glory of our true and perfected human nature and makes relationship with the transcendent world possible; and the darkness that spreads out from the other, which engulfs everything that is good in our human nature and perverts it, cuts off relationship at its root. That difference is everything.

There is a parallel situation with the Holy Scriptures. The Bible is a collection of books, just as a set of mystery stories, or a set of encyclopedias, or a set of pornographic novels are all collections of books. But the one is holy—that is, it is set apart, dedicated to God—and the others are not. Scripture is more than just writing about God: it communicates and reveals God to us; it participates in what it portrays; it makes relationship possible. Similarly, the holy icons are images set apart and dedicated wholly to God; they communicate Him and participate in what they portray, which enables our relationship with Truth, Goodness, and Love.

And pornography, I believe, must be seen in the light of iconography, because pornography portrays people who are made in the image of God—that is, God made them, as He made all of us, to be holy icons. And no matter how badly that icon has been defaced and degraded, while the person still lives, the image is not yet completely destroyed: it remains there to be venerated. If I were purified to illumination, when faced with pornography, I would see there a defaced and degraded image of God. I would still be able to make out amid the grime the true image, and I should venerate that image of God in that person, relating through the veil. But with my impure eye, I am more likely to give my attention to the grime or the masks and abandon myself to my baser desires to abuse the image by objectifying the person.

Saint Nonnus was a monk who had reached a stage of illumination that enabled him to see beyond these masks. Having been taken from his desert monastery and made a bishop on account of his holiness, he was speaking to other bishops at a council in Antioch when a scantily clad actress rode by. The other bishops averted their eyes, but after she had passed, they noticed that St. Nonnus had not only been looking on but was still gazing at her as she disappeared into the distance. They observed him silently and wondered why he had followed this sight rather than averting his eyes as they had. But he said to them, "Did not her great beauty delight you? Indeed, it delighted me."[3] With a purified eye of the heart, why indeed would he want to look away when such a wonder of the beauty of God's creation appeared before his physical eyes? His natural reaction was to delight in the sight and give thanks to God for her. This holy monk looked on the beautiful woman, and in her beauty, he also saw God's: the veneration he directed to the icon passed to the archetype.

I am not holy enough to act as St. Nonnus did; like the other bishops, I need to avert my eyes. But I must be aware that this is because of my passions. If I could be purified and illumined in the way St. Nonnus was, I would be able to properly venerate the image of God in any other human person without inflaming my passions. Yes, without the fullness of purification and illumination, I must avert my eyes, because what I pay to the image—veneration or abuse—has a real impact on relationship, either building up communion or destroying it.

Just as the veneration of an icon passes to its archetype, that link can also be used in the opposite way. For example, in curses and black magic, effigies or images are used to inflict hurt on the archetype in a kind of abusive anti-veneration. Similarly, when I look on another

---

3   Ward, *Harlots*, 59. The veneration with which St. Nonnus looked on the woman also had another effect. He spoke of her beauty while preaching the next day, saying that she took such care to make her body beautiful for her admirers, and this had challenged him to wonder why he had not worked as hard to make his own soul more beautiful for the true Bridegroom. She heard his preaching, was baptized, and is now known as St. Pelagia.

person for my lustful purpose, I direct my evil thoughts outside myself and connect them with another. Since every person is an icon of Christ, this means that the man, woman, or child I see in a pornographic image is an icon of Christ. When I direct lust toward this person, I direct it to Christ Himself.

Can we even imagine being so desensitized that, seeing an icon of Christ, we could experience Him as an object for lust? This seems to be what happened to the men of Sodom (Gen. 19). Two angels (two of the three angels of the Old Testament Trinity icon, which we may assume to be the icons of the Son and the Spirit) went to Sodom, and the men of Sodom saw them as desirable objects for sexual conquest. The angels responded by striking the men blind—that is, by showing physically (symbolically and iconologically) the blindness the men exhibited when they saw Christ and the Holy Spirit as objects of sexual lust. Saint Paul later described this kind of blindness as the darkening of the heart that prevents us from seeing the invisible things of God iconologically in His creation (Rom. 1:19–21).

Veneration, in contrast, relates us to the eschatological truth of the person rather than the sinful immediacy. When we venerate the image of God in each person, we do not venerate the fleshly shadow (the fallenness, brokenness, and sin), just as when we venerate the icon, the purpose is not to bow down to wood and paint. No, when we venerate an icon, it is to us a window through which we can see the prototype: through the icon, we relate. We can gaze into the face of the saint the icon portrays as he or she gazes into us.

The saint is present in the icon, and that presence spills into the world alongside. We are present in the world alongside the icon, and by uniting ourselves in prayer with the saint, we begin to be present in the world of the icon also. And as the saint prays for us, our prayers with and through the saint's are united with the ongoing divine act of remembering that gives us life and makes our presence reality. Likewise, to venerate the image of God in any human person is to encounter something of the fullness of the glorified, ultimate truth of that person as God created him or her to be, and at the same time to look into the eyes of Christ and feel His presence. When we bow down to an icon, we bow to the glorified saint; so we also bow to the one in whose image that saint is made. Likewise, we naturally venerate and bow to those who gain our love and respect—saints, elders, great spiritual fathers and mothers—as they powerfully reveal to us something of the likeness of God. The more perfect the likeness of the image, the more clearly we can see, but that same image itself is present in every human person.

When we relate to our neighbors or any human person as an icon of Christ, when we venerate them, we do not pretend that their imperfections are not there, just as we do not pretend the wood and paint are not there in the icon. We know the imperfections are there, but we also know that they do not define the icon. We know, rather, that the ultimate truth—the real relationship—is with the archetype, the deeper reality beyond the image. With a person, that deeper reality is the eschatological truth of the person—the person we hope to meet in the Kingdom and love for all eternity. To know that there is so much more beyond the field of our vision—that is part of what veneration is about, and the practice of that awareness helps us to avoid abusing the image of God, not only in pornography but in all our everyday relationships.

When we venerate the image of God in another person, we are able to dimly perceive the beautiful fullness of who God created that person to be, rather than seeing the person through assumptions that may have no ground in reality. (Assumptions see a person in the light of a fantasy rather than the light of reality.) Veneration perceives with love. And perceiving with love is not the same as wearing rose-colored glasses; we are not imagining that the wood and paint—the imperfections—are not present. We perceive with love because love is the only way to truly know, relate, and understand. And love is also a barometer of how much we see the person as an icon rather than as a mask based on our own subconscious fantasies about the person and his or her life.

So as we look on the icon of Christ that is every person we meet and every person we see portrayed in photograph, digital image, or video, let us cry, as in the hymn on the Sunday of Orthodoxy—as we claim to cry when we venerate any icon:

O all ye works of the Lord, bless ye the Lord.[4]

---

4   Canticle 8 of the Canon at Matins on the Sunday of Orthodoxy. *Triodion*, 308.

CHAPTER 11

Vulnerability

A T THE END OF CHAPTER 9, I described how standing in front of an icon and praying is an opportunity to open myself and lift my mask in order to be seen, and that to do this is to find myself in a liminal space between presence and absence: I can connect with the saint in the icon, but I cannot yet step fully into the world in which the saint dwells. In the previous chapter, I said that to venerate implies my awareness of this gap—that there is much I still cannot see and cannot know. To open myself up to be seen and known even though I am still unseeing and unknowing is a risk—precisely the risk my masks are designed to protect me from. But protecting myself behind my masks precludes the possibility of real, transformational relationship.

Veils, however, while still permitting my modesty, open a channel for real love and relationship to flow. But they also require me to let go of my attempts at self-preservation and show my vulnerability. If I were to remove the shiny surface of my masks, I would be left with the shadowy layer beneath—the layer of my sin laid bare. Self-examination and the guidance of a spiritual father help me to turn this shadowy layer of the mask into a veil.

Constantine Yiannitsiotis, in his book of reminiscences about his time with St. Porphyrios, illustrates this, describing a time he had tried to reveal something of his desires to the elder.[1] He was "disappointed . . . and somewhat bitter" that the elder had not paid enough attention to his "self-analysis." The elder said to him, "You were sitting here and talking to me and telling me all the holy stuff you wanted to do," but while he was talking, the elder had actually seen "the opposite" and asked him to "think a lot deeper, look right down" into his soul. After praying silently, he confessed, "Elder, you were right. Those things that I said I wanted can be found on the shiny surface of my soul, but what I feel emerging from the depths, is all dark, sinful, and it terrifies me." The elder reassured him, "Don't worry; however, it needs a lot of work."

Once the shiny surface of a mask is lifted through self-examination and support, the shadowy layer below becomes a veil that can start to reveal to me what is really going on deeper within. Without self-examination, I am self-obsessed as, not understanding or knowing what I am doing, I rush to find the climax, to sate my hunger, to fill my needy emptiness. But these shadows, these unconscious drives and desires of mine are veiled truths—not so much about my "individual" being (if such a thing could be said to exist) as about my relational being. As we have seen, all our encounters and interactions constantly change us: we are vulnerable from the beginning—and this is by design. But of course, vulnerability by definition comes with many risks, and I learn to try to protect myself from those risks by closing the entry points—by covering my veils with masks, as Adam and Eve covered their bodies and hid themselves when they realized they were naked (Gen. 3).

But to lock myself behind masks and hide within is to die. We see this in the etymology of the English word *idiot*, which comes from

---

1   Yiannitsiotis, *With Elder Porphyrios*, 41–42.

the Greek ἰδιώτης, (*idiotes*). The primary meaning of the Greek word is the *individual* who does not become involved in communal life— the one who is cut off from relationship and therefore lives a life of ever-decreasing meaning. To be primarily an *individual* is to be cut off; to be fully a *person* is to relate. To fully live is to be vulnerable and respond to the vulnerability of others. It is to enter the conversation, the dynamic of relationship, where everything I offer has meaning and is returned to me transformed. These transformed gifts I receive in turn affect and change me.

This is the path of transformation in an upward spiral of sanctification. It is an iconological reflection of our relationship with God. The clearest example is the case of the Holy Gifts. God provides the seed to us; we receive it and change it by planting it in His earth. God, in turn, sends the rain and sun, so the seed is transformed into wheat and grapes; we harvest and transform them into bread and wine to offer them back to God in the Liturgy. God changes them into the Body and Blood of Christ and offers them back to us; we consume the Gifts, and this feeds and grows our lives. We offer our transformed lives back to God, who in turn offers us life eternal and participation in the divine nature.

However, while this natural relational pattern of transformation is accessible to us, it requires our vulnerability. The temptation since the Fall has been to protect ourselves by cutting ourselves off from it. Vladimir Lossky, author of *The Mystical Theology of the Eastern Church*, describes how Adam and Eve before the Fall, even as two distinct whole persons, shared one common life—one flesh together, perfectly united. In the Fall, they became *individuals*, artificially broken apart, which changed their experience of desire and relationship. He explains:

> A person who asserts himself as an individual, and shuts himself up in the limits of his particular nature, far from realizing himself fully

145

becomes impoverished. It is only in renouncing its own possession and giving itself freely, in ceasing to exist for itself that the person finds full expression in the one nature common to all. In giving up its own specific good, it expands infinitely, and is enriched by everything which belongs to all.[2]

To live as an individual is to live under the protection of the mask—a protection that damages the possibility of relationship and prevents me from fulfilling my vocation as a person in relationship. But to live as a person in relationship requires me to acknowledge and accept my vulnerability. Paradoxically, through attempting to protect myself, I gradually kill myself, and only when I voluntarily step out from behind my self-protective masks and allow myself to be vulnerable, seen through the veil, can I find fullness of life.

Even if I am unable or unwilling to step out into life in this way, and I lock myself behind my masks, I still have my desires, which call me to connection. As a person, I cannot fail to desire connection, and I will always try to communicate, even if, from behind a mask, I must find ways to do this that limit vulnerability. Similarly to C. S. Lewis (whom I quoted above in chapter 8), the pediatrician and psychoanalyst Donald Winnicott speculated that this may be one of the reasons people create art—because it provides a way to communicate from behind the protection of the mask. But in order to truly communicate, we need to transform our masks into veils that protect our modesty while allowing us to be truly known. As Winnicott puts it, referring to a child's game of hide-and-seek, "It is a joy to be hidden, but disaster not to be found."[3] There is no joy in hiding behind

---

2   Lossky, *Mystical Theology*, 123–124.
3   "Here is a picture of a child establishing a private self that is not communicating, and at the same time wanting to communicate and to be found. It is a sophisticated game of hide-and-seek in which it is joy to be hidden but disaster not to be found." Winnicott, *Maturational Processes*, 185.

the mask, but there is a joy in looking out through the veil. The joy occurs when we experience our unique personhood, and this joy is fulfilled when our desire enables us to overcome the fear of our vulnerability and artificial separation, and allow ourselves to be found. Through the veil, desire brings us to encounter, to connection, and to the possibility of change and transformation. And all desire is at the last fulfilled in the joyful true knowledge of (which means *union with*, not *knowledge about*) God.

Meditating on St. Augustine's writing about love, Hannah Arendt describes how desire overcomes separation. Desire, she says,

> annihilates the distance between them by transforming the subject into a lover and the object into the beloved. For the lover is never isolated from what he loves; he belongs to it. . . . Since man is not self-sufficient and therefore always desires something outside himself, the question of who he is can only be resolved by the object of his desire and not, as the Stoics thought, by the suppression of the impulse of desire itself. . . . Strictly speaking, he who does not love and desire at all is a nobody. . . . Man as such, his essence, cannot be defined because he always desires to belong to something outside himself and changes accordingly. . . . If he could be said to have an essential nature at all, it would be lack of self-sufficiency. Hence, he is driven to break out of his isolation by means of love.[4]

But if I am not self-sufficient, if I need others, this is vulnerability and uncertainty, because other whole persons in their own reality will never be entirely predictable and safe for me. I will need to be willing to let go of my own narrative—the story I tell myself about myself—because once I come into connection with another person in all their reality, my story will change. I will no longer have total

4   Arendt, *Love*, 42.

control of my story, and I will not know exactly where I am going. This not knowing, or *unknowing*, in Greek is *agnosia* (the root of the English word *agnostic*), and it is an Orthodox virtue, an essential part of apophatic theology.[5] Openness to reality and to relationship requires *agnosia*—unknowing. Honest, open relationship wherein I am willing to live with the unknowing is dynamic, life-giving; it will reveal the truth about me and will also allow me to take steps toward the real fulfillment of my desire, rather than settling for a temporary satiety. The alternative to unknowing is certainty; the alternative to dynamic unpredictability is predictability or stasis—standing still and never growing or developing. And the only total certainty in this life is death.

But there are things about myself that I do not want to know. This is not the same as *agnosia* because in this case, on a deeper, subconscious level, these are things I do know, but I wish not to know, and therefore, the masks that my subconscious creates to protect me will not allow me to know. These things I have hidden from myself result in my most convincing masks, as I myself in my conscious mind do not realize they are lies. Because of this, the things I don't want to know about myself will manifest in my greatest struggles. The temptations are the masks that cover the reality—they are the way I subconsciously hide it even from myself.

I hide things from myself for many reasons, but in general, they often connect in some way to past trauma, to something or things that have happened to me that I am unable to cope with. The memory is unbearable, and therefore I refuse to allow myself to know or remember it. I cannot allow myself to be vulnerable to these things, because I feel certain that I could not go on living with myself in a life where these things were true.

---

5   The theological path that avoids making specific statements about God on the basis that all human language is inadequate to express anything ultimately true of God, who is essentially unknowable and ineffable.

Alternatively, or in addition to this, it may be that I do not want to know what my deeper desires are for fear that I cannot find a way to meet them. Or perhaps I fear that if I allowed myself to feel my deeper desire, it would lead me to certain death and destruction. So the temptations that form the shadowy layer of my mask present me with a desire for something attainable instead—for example, pornography. But since my mask hides my real desire, it prevents me from fulfilling it. The mask presents only a superficial fulfillment, which is ultimately not satisfying, so the temptation will return again and again; in my inability to be vulnerable, my deeper, more authentic desire is never met. All my appetites are frightening. I desperately try to control them because my desires lead to connections in unpredictable and uncontrollable ways. But because these desires are the protective masks over my real desires, my ability to control them is limited, and I will continually fail.

I have been describing these temptations, these desires, as the shadowy layer of the masks. But once the shiny top layer of a mask has been stripped away, it is apparent that this shadowy underlayer is now a veil. Without the cover of the brightly painted surface, it is much easier for me to see through the shadows—the veil—and detect my real self underneath. But only if I am able to be vulnerable.

So if I am addicted to pornography (or indeed, to any other behavior aimed at meeting these superficial desires), I may find it is not so much the porn that is the problem as the vulnerability I am trying to protect by using porn. And it is not so much a problem to be solved as it is a *fact* of this life that needs to be transformed into the *truth* beyond the veil. The pornography hides the vulnerability, soothes the pain, mitigates the suffering, plasters over the need, obviates the necessity of grieving. But once I see it is the shadowy layer of the mask of desire and understand that, the mask loses its power to misdirect me. It therefore becomes a veil that reveals my true desire and opens a path to transformation.

This way, I begin to see through the veil by accepting my real vulnerability, and thereby I am able to access my deeper desire. However deep I go, I will find desire. Desire is what enables me to step outside my individual existence into a relational personhood. Desire is at the heart of life, so I fear its loss. But I also fear its power. This is why I am tempted by these middling desires, the shadowy protective desires of my masks—desires that are strong enough to let me know I am still alive but that are relatively safe and superficial, not making me more vulnerable than I can handle. It is safer to lose myself for a while in porn because I know where that desire ends, and after that, I can return to my everyday life. But it is unsafe to reveal myself and my vulnerability through my veil to another person. In the same way, it is wholly unsafe to lose myself mystically in prayer before an icon. Both things are unsafe, because once I allow that deeper access to myself through the veil, I have no idea where my desire ends or what it means for my life.

One person I know, when praying before the icon of Christ to overcome his addictive behaviors, asked God to bless him by opening his desires for good instead of for these petty evils, and to connect him to the real world rather than his own fantasy world. Afterward, he said, it was difficult for him to function in everyday life for a while. At one point, shortly after praying this way, he went to pick up a cup, and its beauty overwhelmed him. The texture and weight of it were so significant that it was hard for him to let go of it. For a while, the beauty of everything he saw and touched filled him with such an intensity of feeling and appreciation that he was physically almost overwhelmed. The feeling faded after a while, but perhaps it was an intimation of the fullness of life beyond the veil. Or perhaps his protective shadowy desires had cut him off from real, deep feeling for so long that once he was able to step through the veil into his real vulnerability and reveal his deeper desire before Christ present in the icon, the access to the reality of his deeper feelings became overwhelming in its intensity. And perhaps both of these possibilities are an expression of the same reality.

One of the significant aspects of the experience related above was its dispassionate nature. The feelings were intense, but not in the same way that lust is intense, weighted with passion. In the Orthodox understanding, the passions are aspects of our experience that reduce us to a state of passivity or slavery, overcoming our will and our deeper desire.[6] This is what I have been describing as the shadowy layer of the masks. The passions manifest in us those desires that, no matter how much we indulge them, can never fulfill us.

It is no wonder that this particular experience of dispassionate love for God's creation described above followed a period of intense prayer in front of an icon, because the icon is dispassionate by design. Unlike many other forms of art and imagery, icons are specifically designed not to arouse the passions and emotions, precisely because icons are veils of ultimate truth and perfect relationship: they are windows to the place where the deeper desires can truly be fulfilled. Pornographic imagery, in contrast, arouses the passions, both in the moment of use and in its general effects, and the passions mask the truth of my condition. The more we learn to see through the veil (or in other words, the closer we are to real relationship, in full acceptance of our real selves and our vulnerability), the less active our defensive passions will be, and the closer we will be able to get to dispassion.

Dispassion can be differentiated from *detachment*, although from the outside they may sometimes appear similar.[7] To make a clear distinction, I will use the word *detachment* to mean the preservation of the individualistic autonomy of my life at the expense of real living and relating. In contrast, *dispassion* (usually achieved only through

---

6   This point and the next one are the two key points Staniloae begins with in his introduction to the passions in *Orthodox Spirituality*, 77–83.

7   The word *detachment* is also used in many texts in the sense that I am using *dispassion*. Context will determine the meaning.

long ascetic practice) would permit me to truly live and relate in full awareness of my reality and the reality of the other without losing control of my emotional reactions. The fuller form of detachment is *dissociation*—in which I cut off my internal reality from my external reality. Dissociation is a psychological condition which usually arises as a result of overwhelming trauma or torture—when the only way to protect myself from what is happening to me (over which I have no control) is to subconsciously disconnect my internal life more or less completely from external reality. Dissociation is an almost universal experience for those working in prostitution and pornography[8] because of the trauma this involves for the people concerned.

Dissociation, then, is disappearing completely behind my mask, from where I can make no real contact with others and where the world outside can no longer reach me. And as I have said, to stay behind my masks, cutting myself off from the world and the possibility of relationship in an unchanging individualism, is in the end death. Simone Weil identified this in her famous comment that there are "two ways of killing ourselves: suicide or detachment."[9] This contrast between dispassion and detachment again illustrates the Lord's saying that those who try to save their lives will lose them, but those who are willing to risk their lives for the sake of the Way, the Truth, and the Life will find life in greater fullness.

This contrast between finding life through dispassion and losing it through detachment is illustrated in the life of Iulia de Beausobre, a Russian noblewoman tortured by the GPU (a predecessor of the KGB in the Soviet Union). She spent many years in the gulag and wrote about her experience of torture in a memoir published after she escaped the USSR in the 1930s. She was tempted toward detachment and dissociation (which, she says, lead to madness). But

---

8   Moran, *Paid For*, 138–150.
9   Weil, *Gravity and Grace*, 15.

in Christ (beginning even before she had consciously realized that it was Christ whose presence she felt) she learned rather to connect dispassionately to the full reality of everything going on around her, including in empathy toward her torturers themselves. Detachment, on the other hand, enables torturers to do their work.[10] The Nazi Heinrich Himmler said, "To have stuck it out and, apart from exceptions caused by human weakness, to have remained decent, that is what has made us hard."[11] This hardness, or detachment, may appear civilized and "decent" on the surface, in the right context—but it is actually the shiny surface of a mask covering a whole array of unseen demonic passions.

Vulnerability is the opposite of detachment: vulnerability is involvement. Full involvement in life is risky and sometimes painful, but it is also the only path by which we can arrive at true joy. Life can be torturous, but the way of Gethsemane is "Thy will, not mine, be done" (Luke 22:42). This prayer releases us into the fullness of life through our vulnerability as we gradually learn that we can indeed trust God's will, and that although we may be led into the valley of the shadow of death, He will always be with us. This life is, in fact, the valley of the shadow of death. It is by definition a liminal place: the threshold of eternity, the boundary between heaven and hell, the place of possibility and potential. To live is therefore to be vulnerable, always potentially at the mercy of others, and always at the mercy of death.

In this life, I sit in this liminal place, and I may feel that my desire is all-consuming; there seems no way for me to meet it. This is a different kind of torture from the one inflicted by the GPU, but both

---

10 In her autobiography, *The Woman Who Could Not Die*. She described some of her reflections on her experience in a talk titled "Creative Suffering" that she gave in London in the 1940s, which is still available in a booklet by the same name.

11 Quoted in Arendt, *Eichmann*, 103.

indicate that in this life we are on the very edge of both heaven and hell. Hell is that endless unfulfilled desire, that torture of seeing but never being seen, hearing but never being heard, reaching out but never being met. Descending into hell is torture, but if I can accept my vulnerability and allow myself to be truly involved in the experience, it is a fire that can burn away all my masks and open me again to the possibility of real relationship and of grace. But how can I spend time in this hell without despair? In despair, I cannot hope that the pain of this moment will eventually be over, and so I turn again to my soothing coping behaviors, such as pornography use or fantasies of various kinds, and attempt to avoid the suffering of this place of unknowing, of loneliness, of driving need. But as I sit in this place, I hear the voice of St. Silouan: "Keep your mind in hell and despair not."[12]

I mentioned above the experience of Iulia de Beausobre under torture. This unfulfilled desire, this place of being unseen and unheard, is my torture. Can I learn from the approach she was enabled to practice under much more severe and painful conditions? To keep my mind in hell—to open myself to all the fullness of the suffering of the world—would require limitless humility, courage, and strength, none of which I have. How could I not despair? Christ, however, has all these things, as we see in the story of His Passion and death. If we can truly dwell in the love of Christ, we will be able to access these things, and therefore we will be able to keep our minds in hell and despair not. In other words, as St. Silouan says, "the one who knows 'how greatly the Lord loveth us' escapes the pernicious effect of total despair and knows how to stand prudently *on the verge* so that the hellish fire burns away his every passion and he does not fall victim to despair."[13]

---

12   Sophrony, *Saint Silouan*, 208ff.
13   Sophrony, 211.

This place—*on the verge*—is where I need to stand. Failing in my own strength, I look through the veil into the face of Christ and unite myself to His love. I surround myself with goodness and beauty (Phil. 4:8), prayer and communion. I immerse myself in the Church. The Church, the spiritual hospital, is a unique kind of hospital because it is where the sick meet not only the doctors but also the healed (through the icons). There we find communion with other sick people in various stages of healing, along with the medics, the healed, and all the ranks of armies of angels ready to fight for our health, life, and joy.

This experience of standing *on the verge*, of perceiving the reality of hell, is where I reach the end of myself. It is the ultimate vulnerability, where I feel my life is lost, where everything is possible and the fear is past. In this moment, this place, my priorities are completely changed. In this moment I can have total trust in Christ, and there is no reason any longer to hold anything at all back from Him. I can give Him, in tears, all of me, explicitly naming all the abused and defiled parts of me, and it will not be in passion but in peace. This is a blessed place—the place that is the answer to our frequent petition: "From all necessity, O Lord, deliver us."[14] It is the place where I can let go of all needs and simply *be*. And as I release my passionate attachment to my needs, it becomes clear that the appropriate response to every need is not to desire a counterfeit fulfillment. The appropriate response is grief and mourning, because every need is a loss, an absence. Grief and mourning are the proper response to loss. This is also a gradual process of letting go rather than holding on (in obsession or addiction)—a process again of bringing myself into line with reality.

I find the end of myself, like the prodigal son in the pigsty (Luke 15:11–32), when I reach the very bottom. There, I acknowledge in true humility my real condition—and I receive an opportunity to

---

14   Taken from the Great Ektenia (Litany) in the Liturgy of St. John Chrysostom.

find freedom. Total vulnerability feels like weakness, and I may want to pray to be released from all vulnerability and weakness. But in reality, seeing, facing, acknowledging, and knowing my vulnerability is strength, as St. Paul says: "Thrice I called on the Lord about this that it would leave me. And He said to me, 'My grace is enough for you. For My power is perfected in weakness'" (2 Cor. 12:8–9). Opening up the weakness, the vulnerability, stepping into and living it, permits real transformation, because the end of myself is the place where I can finally face my fears, the place where the veil between this world and the next is very thin. I can see down through the veil and look at the dragons in my heart—the dragons that stop me from truly loving. The gift of desperation is that it takes me to that place where my vulnerability is no longer in question. To the pigsty where the pigs' food looks appetizing because I have and am nothing but my fears. And that is why that is the place of true repentance and the starting point from which it is possible to find love.

There in the pigsty, I find true freedom. True freedom is the willingness to lose everything. Without this, there are ties that bind me and limit my ability to act. Unfortunately, that often means that I have to come to a place where I have nothing left to lose before I can exercise true freedom. This is why Jesus said to the rich young ruler, "If you want to be perfect, go and sell what you possess and give to the poor, and you will have treasure in heaven, and come, follow Me" (Matt. 19:21). This freedom enables us to find true joy. When I perceive what lies on the other side of the veil, I can discover what desires I have that lead me to true joy in freedom from all necessity, where I no longer desire something to fill an immediate need. True joy lies here: when I have nothing left to offer, when I get to the end of myself, when I am exposed in total vulnerability, I find that God still loves me. My value lies in nothing I have, nothing I can do, but just in myself.

At the end of myself, I have a real choice: I can turn toward love, I can face and accept what is deep and dark within me and decide to go through it, or I can simply drown in my fears and look on love from the outside as something I can never dwell in. And there is no way to know which I will choose, which I will be able to choose, which I will (in the end) even *want* to choose, until that moment when I make my choice—or until I make a choice by choosing not to move at all, through inertia or despair. But I have at least some time: as long as I live, the possibility of returning to my Father's house and His love and His feast is always open.

A Prayer of Return[15]

Open Thine arms, O Christ,
and in loving-kindness receive me
as I return from a far country of sin and passions.
(See color photo insert D.)

---

15   From the Matins Canon on the Sunday of the Prodigal Son. *Triodion*, 116.

CHAPTER 12

Freedom

I N THE PREVIOUS CHAPTER, WE saw that we find freedom in
acknowledging our vulnerability by allowing ourselves to be seen
through the veil. Until we learn to do this, the passions—the masks—
hold us in a state of passivity and slavery. Jesus said, "Everyone who
practices sin is a slave of sin" (John 8:34). This is true of all sin, and we
have seen in our discussion of pornography how easy it is to become a
slave of sexual sin. And we have seen specifically how that slavery eats
away at our freedom, and at the same time increasingly degrades and
destroys the likeness of God in us. We know, though, that the image
of God in which we are made is never destroyed, because so long as
we live, we live only through God's dynamic, life-sustaining power
active in us.

Many of the ascetic Fathers talk about this slavery to sin and how
we can seek freedom in Christ. The best-known of the Desert Fathers,
St. Anthony the Great, tells us:

A man is free if he is not a slave to sensual pleasures, but through good
judgment and self-restraint masters the body and with true gratitude
is satisfied with what God gives him, even if it is quite scanty. If the

158

soul and the [*nous*] that enjoys the love of God are in harmony, the whole body is peaceful even against its wishes.[1]

Saint Anthony also points out that freedom is not something that can be provided from outside, nor something we can attain by power; it is something we develop inside ourselves through inner communion with God in Christ:

Regard as free not those whose status makes them outwardly free, but those who are free in their character and conduct. For we should not call men in authority truly free when they are wicked or dissolute, since they are slaves to worldly passions. Freedom and happiness of soul consist in genuine purity and detachment from transitory things.[2]

Saint Paul also emphasizes the point that we can find true freedom only in communion with Christ—that is, by receiving Christ into ourselves (Gal. 2:20) and by putting on Christ as our garment (Rom. 13:14). This is the way we can begin living in harmony with the image of God in which we are made. This is how we start finding the freedom to live in the image of God, as St. Paul explains: "Having taken off the old self with its practices and put on the new," we are "being renewed into an acknowledgement of the Creator's image" (Col. 3:9–10). This is a description of how putting away our masks allows us to know and be known through the veil.

Those of us who have struggled and continue to struggle with sexual sin and temptations to sexual sin have experienced just how

---

1   "On the Character of Men," 56, in *Philokalia* Vol. 1, 337.
2   "On the Character of Men," 18, *Philokalia* Vol. 1, 332. "Detachment," in the sense it is used here, is not the isolating, individualist detachment from creation I spoke of in the previous chapter, but a dispassion and the refusal to unite ourselves with the flesh, the body of death.

that sin is slavery, but we have also at least had glimpses of the free-dom Christ offers through union with Him. But I want to look at this picture now from the other side. What about those of us who do not believe that we have a particular problem with sexual sin—who think we are free from slavery to these desires? Of course, we all have the odd temptation, but many of us habitually stand strong and yet have much sympathy for those who find this so difficult. We want to find ways to help people who struggle with sexual sin to find strength in their struggles. How do we help them?

In the early twentieth century, an Austrian Catholic apologist, the Baron von Hügel, wrote approvingly about a nun who was deeply concerned for one of her former pupils from the convent school.[3] After leaving the school, this young woman had become the lover of a wealthy man in town. The nun knew by experience that she could not argue her protégée out of her decisions about the life she was leading, whether by appealing to religion, or to conscience, or even to her own good in the long term. This nun, in other words, was in exactly the sit-uation I outlined above—the situation many of us may find ourselves in, where someone we care about is living a life that we know to be at the very least spiritually unhealthy and dangerous. We want to help them change. What do we do when argument makes no difference? When we pray, and yet nothing seems to change? When we see the person we care about slipping away from us into this other life that is so far from Christ, so far from everything they have been taught in the Church and have previously professed?

This nun decided there was one more path she could take—a self-sacrificial path out of love for this young woman, a way to make her friend feel that the lifestyle she had fallen into was wrong. So she wrote to her, saying that she knew her young friend cared for her

---

3   Hügel, *Essays & Addresses,* 240–41, also discussed by de Beausobre in *Creative Suffering.*

and wanted her to live to a ripe old age. The nun went on to say that every day the friend continued to live in this immoral lifestyle, "she, the nun, would scourge herself until her feet stood in a pool of her own blood."[4] She wrote to her friend that she had already started to put this plan into action, and nothing would stop her until her young friend confirmed that she had changed her course and left her sexual immorality behind. After a few days, the nun received a letter from her young friend, telling her that the nun had succeeded in her attempt—the young woman had broken off the relationship. But what, in reality, had this nun achieved?

At the beginning of this chapter, I quoted the Lord saying, "Everyone who practices sin is a slave of sin" (John 8:34). A little earlier in the same chapter of St. John's Gospel, we find the story of the woman caught in adultery (John 8:3–11), which we can compare to the story of the nun and her young friend above. Like the young friend of the nun, this woman had fallen into sexual immorality. The Lord cared about her deeply, just as the nun cared about her young friend. Although she did not face a stoning like the woman in the Gospel account, the nun's young friend in the early twentieth century certainly faced social disapproval and other worldly condemnations of her behavior.

But Jesus did something different from the nun. He challenged the accusers to look at their own hearts, and when they did so, they found that perhaps they were not in so strong a position as they had thought they were, in comparison to the woman caught in adultery. So they slipped away quietly. And Jesus said, "Where are they? Did none of them condemn you?" adding, "Neither do I condemn you. Go on your way! And from now on, sin no more!" (John 8:10–11). The Lord does not condemn, does not emotionally blackmail, give a sermon, or talk of consequences, does not bewail lost innocence or talk of

---

4   Hügel, 241.

falling away. None of this. Instead, He simply utters three short sentences. With the first, "Neither do I condemn you!" we learn that it is not condemnation that will inspire repentance. And with the simple imperative, "Go on your way!" Jesus affirms the woman's—and our—freedom. He does not force us to do good but waits for us in our freedom to choose the path of love and righteousness. The pressures may be great; there may be all kinds of good reasons that lead us into any given situation; nevertheless, the woman, like the rest of us, does have some choice. We all have our freedom—limited, and yet still present. But while He does not force the woman to change, Jesus does issue a strong and direct call to repentance: "And from now on, sin no more!"

In the light of this example, we can see where the nun in the story above went wrong. She loved the young woman deeply and wanted all good for her, but with the best of motives, she *forced* the woman to do the right thing. And by forcing her, she prevented the young woman from *choosing* to do the right thing. She took away the young woman's freedom, and in so doing, took away her ability to love. She took away her ability to repent. Instead of encouraging the young woman to understand her own actions, to examine her heart and her mask, to perceive through the veil what was going on within and then in freedom to submit herself to Christ, she forced her friend to submit to herself, to her own threats, her own emotional blackmail. She took away the possibility of the great joy the young woman could have found by freely following Him who simply said, "Go on your way! And . . . sin no more!" Without freedom, love and true repentance are impossible. These two things are the same thing, of course, because true repentance involves opening ourselves in love of God—a willingness to throw ourselves into the open arms of Christ.

So how do we help? We first have to realize that we are part of the crowd Jesus spoke to in this story. We may not be lining up with literal stones to throw, but what are we offering? If we do not have self-knowledge and self-awareness enough to see what we are doing, we will offer the brightly painted shiny surface of a hardened and impenetrable mask. To the vulnerable person who has begun to lift the protection of their own mask, our well-intentioned, superficial desire to make things better may turn out to be just another stone.

Before we are ready to help others, we must look inside ourselves in order to detect our own masks and find our own freedom, and in so doing, realize that we have been seeing those people we want to help as masks rather than as people like us. We have not truly loved them or desired their freedom, but rather, we have desired that they should change their masks to masks more like our own. We see that there is not a meaningful difference between us—all have sinned and fallen short of the glory of God (Rom. 3:23). We all reflect something of the image of God, and yet none of us, in the darkened mirrors of our lives, reflect the glory of His likeness. All of us have our masks and are called to learn to see through the veils in order to love our neighbor as ourselves.

So whether we struggle with sexual sin ourselves or want to help others who have to some degree formed their lives in a context of sexual sin, let us be aware that there is no repentance without love and freedom. Although at times we use force on ourselves (the force of the ascetic path, for example, against our desires for bodily plea-sure), this is a force born of freedom and love, and we choose it for ourselves; it is not forced on us from outside. We choose to exercise restraint because we desire to conform ourselves to Christ's life and live in union with Him. The path is hard, my soul is weak, and I choose to exercise force on myself because a significant part of me does not want to choose love, does not want to turn over my freedom to God. A part of me does not want to really understand and come to know what lies beneath the veil, because I fear I could not love it— what lies behind the veil (the real me) may actually be unlovable.

And yet, even the violence I practice against the passions is not going to win me salvation! That can come only through the grace of God, through union with Christ in His Crucifixion and Resurrection. And while we cannot force those around us to exercise their freedom in this way, what we can do is inspire them with the love of Christ, so that they will choose to do those things in and of themselves, with God's help and ours.

Let's keep in mind that freedom is a double-edged sword, however. Without freedom, I cannot truly love God or neighbor. Without freedom, I cannot truly repent. Without freedom, I cannot turn myself over to holiness in choosing to be a slave to Christ. But it is also in my freedom that I fall into sin, that I follow my passions, that I make myself a slave to demons. The difference, of course, is that in becoming slaves to Christ we find perfect freedom, because in union with Christ we can become fully ourselves, the person we were created to be—as behind the veil we truly are images of God. But in becoming a slave to demons, although I seem to be following my own desires in my own way, I lose all freedom, and I form myself, in cooperation with the demons, into something much less than a person.

Sexual sin is a clear manifestation of slavery, because it is a particularly clear manifestation of the union my desires move me toward. If I fall deeply enough into sexual sin, I will see where it leads at the point where I am faced with my own destruction. I see how seeking union with anything or anyone outside of and apart from God and truth gradually takes away my freedom, my personhood, my ability to be uniquely myself. The further I fall, the more I am corrupted, and the clearer my anti-iconological idolatry becomes. The further I fall, the more I need to exercise that violence, that force against my passions and desires—the dark desires deep in my soul—in order to repent. And yet, the further I fall, the less I am able to exercise that force, as my freedom to choose is damaged more and more.

The loss of freedom in relation to sexuality is particularly acute because physical sexuality is a symbol—that is, both an image and a physical manifestation—of union. In marriage, our physical union with our spouse is to be an icon of the Church's spiritual union with God in Christ (Eph. 5:31–32). In this union, we see how our love for God and our love for our closest neighbor is one love. In any real union—whenever we genuinely open ourselves to the other and meet them through our veils—we become more and more like those with whom we unite ourselves. In union with God, we become more godly. In union with Christ, we take on the attributes of Christlikeness. This is perfect love, perfect freedom, the ability to be who we are, who we were created to be.

But in any union that requires me to be apart from Christ, I begin to lose all those things, because physical sexuality misdirected—however it is misdirected—is an image of disintegration. Not only does it distance me from Christ, as I seek union outside and apart from Him, but it also heralds my disintegration as a person. I am practicing a union with that which can never give me true freedom, a union that will never allow me to become truly myself, a union with that which, ultimately, is just nothingness.

As I go further and further into any pattern of life, any kind of relationship—as I begin to unite myself with anything in creation—I can examine myself in order to discern whether this is leading me through the veil toward Christ or away from Him toward nothingness: Are my desires turning me more and more toward love? Or are they turning me more and more toward isolation? Is my freedom growing, enabling me more often to choose the good, to choose love of God and neighbor, to see beyond the veil? Or is my freedom gradually closing down, leading me to seem to have no choice in continuing the path I chose long ago, leading me to addiction, slavery to sin, and ever more brightly painted masks to obscure the shadows beneath? Am I becoming more myself—am I growing in love for God and neighbor? Am I able to stand freely even in the face of disapproval from others, in the face of persecution—can I stand for what I believe in even unto death? Or am I losing the strength to be myself—am I painting my mask in conformity with the masks of those I have chosen to live among, even when I would rather do otherwise? Can I see beyond the shiny surface of my soul to the darkness that lurks beneath? Can I be honest with myself about the desires that lie inside?

While I have life, there is something of the image of God left in me, however tarnished the likeness to God may be. I may have acted in such a way, or lived in such a context, or I may be so severely traumatized that over time my ability to exercise my freedom is decreased and damaged. But as the saying goes, while there is life, there is hope. Repentance can begin at any moment. So while I have life, I still have some freedom left. Can I use that freedom to turn to Christ, to turn away from all demonic desires that will define me if I do not turn away?

I cannot do it alone, that is certain; I do not have that sort of strength. But I can turn to the Church, to the Mysteries of the Church. I can confess the darkness in my soul and ask for help. I can receive Christ in the Holy Mysteries and live into holiness by seeking out holy people who will help me, and asking for their prayers and the prayers of the saints. None of this is easy, but through it joy will come, and grace will be given. It is a burden to be yoked to Christ, to be united with Him, but as Christ said, "My yoke is easy and my burden is light" (Matt. 11:30). Saint Porphyrios confirms this too, saying, "Many say that the Christian Life is disagreeable and difficult; I say that it is agreeable and easy, but it requires two preconditions: humility and love."[5] In whatever remains of our freedom, can we choose humility and love?

---

5   Yiannitsiotis, *Elder Porphyrios*, 50.

A Prayer of Freedom[6]

As of old Thou didst redeem us from the curse of the law
by Thy Divine-flowing Blood, O Jesus,
likewise rescue us from the snares in which the serpent hath entangled us
through the passions of the flesh,
through lustful suggestions,
and evil despondency,
as we cry unto Thee: Alleluia!

---

6   Kontakion 5 from the Akathist to Our Sweetest Lord Jesus Christ.
     Akathists, 36.

CHAPTER 13

My Wedding Garment

V EILS, OF COURSE, ARE STRONGLY associated with marriage; the veil is a symbol of union and the possibility of union. In contrast, the mask, representing sin and separation, is a symbol of play-acting, of deception, and of unfaithfulness—itself the characteristic symbol of immorality. To talk about unfaithfulness (*porneia*) is to talk in reference to marriage, and marriage as an icon is absolutely central to our faith.

Marriage is at the heart of everything from the beginning of humanity to the end of the world. At the Creation of humanity as male and female, the Holy Scripture immediately makes reference to marriage (Gen. 2:23–25), and Christ refers back to this passage explicitly when He speaks of marriage (Matt. 19:5). The relationship between God and Israel is described in the Old Testament as marriage,[1] and the relationship between Christ and His Church is described as marriage in the New. Israel's straying from God is characterized as adultery,[2] and when Israel returns, this is God recon-

---

1   For example, Ezek. 16:1–15 describes the love story of when Israel first
     encounters God. See also Is. 54:5; Jer. 2:2; and the story of Hosea.
2   For example, Ezek. 16:15–34; Jer. 3:20.

ciling with His bride.[3] Christ is the Bridegroom of the Church[4] (see color photo insert E), and St. Paul speaks of marriage as a great mystery in terms of the union of Christ and the Church (Eph. 5:25–33). Finally, the Holy Bible ends with the marriage feast of the Lamb (Rev. 19:6–9; 21:1–9).

This is not to say that every one of us is called to find a husband or wife. On the contrary, St. Paul makes it clear that this is not true, saying that in many cases it is better to remain single (1 Cor. 7:8–9). But every one of us is called to participate in the mystical marriage that is union with God in Christ. Every time we participate in the Divine Liturgy, we participate in the wedding feast, and this wedding feast is at the heart of all the mysteries of the faith. God calls all people to this marriage, just as in the parable of the wedding banquet (Matt. 22:1–14), people were called in from the highways and byways of the city. All were invited—but in order to take their places at the wedding banquet, they needed to prepare by putting on a wedding garment. What is this wedding garment? It is a veil that reveals who I really am, just as creation as a whole is the veil that reveals who God is. When we don the wedding garment, we prepare to participate fully—body, mind, and spirit—in this union. Saint Gregory of Rome, the Dialogist, says that the wedding garment is a garment of love, woven using the two crossing threads of love for God and love for neighbor. Christ tells us that the whole law depends on these two things (Matt. 22:40) and that we fulfill the law through participating fully in His wedding banquet.[5]

So the wedding feast is starting, and I am invited. Why then don't I put on the wedding garment? Because when it comes down to it, I

---

3   For example, Ezek. 16:59–62 and Is. 62:3–5.
4   John the Baptist first refers to this as such (John 3:28–29). See also Matt. 9:15; 2 Cor. 11:2; and parables such as Matt. 22:1–14/Luke 14:15–24 and Matt. 25:1–13.
5   Homily 38 on the Gospels, Gregory the Great, *Forty Gospel Homilies*, 347.

don't want to participate fully in the marriage that means union with God in Christ. I don't wholeheartedly want what God wants for my life. I want my own way—I want somehow to combine faithfulness to God with the ability to protect myself, to keep my own vulnerability safely hidden. I seek connection and union, but at the same time, I want to protect my vulnerability. And my inability to be truly vulnerable when it gets too hard prevents the true intimacy I desire, causing me to turn to lesser, safer desires.

The whole story of the Old Testament describes this tension between Israel's love for God and her unfaithfulness to Him.[6] Israel seeks union but then loses faith and turns from that union, which asks for total involvement, total vulnerability, and commitment. Instead, Israel seeks lesser unions that do not ask as much but also cannot deliver what they promise. This is characteristic of the porn user too, as we have seen. But it is also the characteristic way of relating for all of us who fail to put on the wedding garment and keep it on always.

So rather than accepting this call to eschatological marriage, or perfect union, I want to find fulfillment with an easier partner— one who does not and cannot really know me. But this is incompatible with my other, deeper desire—to be truly loved for who I really am. And this is what this marital love and union is about: it is truly to *know* and truly to *be known*. Recall that the King James Version of the Bible says, "And Adam *knew* Eve his wife; and she conceived" (Gen. 4:1, my italics). This is not a euphemism; it is a deep truth. This physical act of union, in order to be experienced in its fullness, has to be a manifestation of both a psychological encounter and a spiritual truth—the *knowing* and *being known* happens on the level of body, mind, and spirit. It also bears fruit on all these levels. And a

---

6   The references at the beginning of this chapter are starting points for exploring this story, which the Old Testament covers in both imagery and history. Saint Paul gives a very brief summary in 1 Cor. 10:1–14.

husband's love for his wife is to be an image—an icon—of God's love for all humanity, of Christ's love for His Church. We must love God as a bride loves her bridegroom. The promise is that in the fulfillment of this mystical marriage we will participate in the very life of God—and sexual love in earthly marriage is the most direct physical icon of this ultimate love and union.[7]

The fact that every union functions on all these levels—never only on the physical—is all part of the iconographic way of seeing; these are simply more details about how creation is iconological. We often hear that creation teaches us about God—and this is true—but the reality is much deeper than that. Creation not only teaches us, not only reveals God to us, but it allows—in fact, requires—that we participate in the life of God, either for good or for ill. And the only way we can participate for good is by putting on the wedding garment.

Seeing truly, seeing iconographically and iconologically, is about being in touch with Reality—with God. It means there is an unbreakable link between what goes on in our bodies, in our minds, and in our souls. The physical and the spiritual are intrinsically connected, within creation in general and in the human person in particular. And St. Maximos the Confessor goes even further, referring to the human person using the Hellenic concept of *microcosm*: each person is a "little cosmos," an icon of all creation as well as the image of God. That is to say, a union with God and with all creation is built into our very existence, even though we may turn away from this union in unfaithfulness. And it is by putting on the wedding garment that we live into this deep truth of our very being.

---

7   The direct link between the physical and the spiritual in marriage is clear in the story of Hosea, where the prophet's marriage to a prostitute images the spiritual reality of God's marriage to unfaithful Israel. "When the Lord first spoke through Hosea, the Lord said to Hosea, 'Go, take to yourself a wife of harlotry and have children of harlotry; for the land commits flagrant harlotry, forsaking the Lord'" (Hos. 1:2).

Not seeing iconologically is idolatry, which is unfaithfulness in its most obvious, most characteristic sense. Not seeing God in His creation is not being faithful; it is losing faith, not trusting Him. Pornography is simply one of the most blatant examples of not seeing iconologically, specifically in regard to the human person—that is, specifically in regard to the image of God. To break the iconographic way of seeing is to separate the physical from the spiritual—to objectify the physical, just as using pornography objectifies the person and breaks the link between the physical and spiritual, making true relationship impossible. This form of unfaithfulness is just one example of the unfaithfulness implicit in using creation in any context that excludes relating to God. When we do this, we avoid putting on the wedding garment and therefore miss the chance to participate in the fullness of love.

When it comes down to it, this non-iconographic way of seeing the world is by nature unfaithfulness. When I look at creation and I don't see God, it is like looking at the physical body of a woman in loveless lust and not seeing the fullness of the person. And Jesus said that to look at a woman with lust is to commit adultery in my heart—that is, to be unfaithful. When I look with lust, I also objectify. Lust always means using others to gratify my desires. Even if someone reciprocates my lust, it is not love. Mutual lust is still each seeking his or her own pleasure—it is taking another for myself rather than a mutual self-offering to the other. Even if I lust for my spouse, the same applies. When St. Paul advises those who "burn" with lust to marry (1 Cor. 7:9), it is not because burning with lust is acceptable in marriage, but because marriage is a path that can enable us to transform the desire at the root of that lust into something deeper and fuller. It enables us to see beyond the veil of the physical into deeper spiritual realities, to see iconologically.

It's important to stress again here that God does not call us to cut off desire at the root but to don the wedding garment and join the banquet. Purity is not achieved by killing or suppressing our desires; rather, it allows them to be transformed and redirected toward the possibility of being ultimately satisfied. That is, I find purity when my body properly reflects not the shadowy desires of my mask but the deeper desire of my spirit. In fact, as C. S. Lewis often points out, our desires are not too strong but too weak. He says, "We are half-hearted creatures, fooling about with drink and sex and ambition when infinite joy is offered us," adding that our desires in truth lead us "to taste at the fountainhead that stream of which even these lower reaches prove so intoxicating."[8]

So this desire at the root of lust is not evil, it is just misdirected, disorientated; it misses the mark. And missing the mark, of course, is the definition of sin.[9] The mark is Christ, the true and full human being. Sin is missing Christ—missing the Bridegroom and hitting on someone or something else. So sin, by definition, is unfaithfulness, and specifically, because of our marital union with Christ, sin is marital unfaithfulness. Unfaithfulness, then, is the characteristic act of immorality; whether it is something I do by choice, by enticement and seduction, or even by compulsion, it causes separation from the source of life and love.

Just as unfaithfulness is turning away, learning to be faithful again is turning back; it is the process of repentance. Repentance is the purpose of this life—it prepares me for the life to come. And the life to come is the wedding banquet, which I prepare for by putting on my wedding garment. This is why the wedding garment—the love of God and neighbor—holds in itself all that the law requires. Preparing for participation in the Divine Liturgy by confession and reconciliation to God and neighbor is an icon of this same process. And in this process of repentance in love, of donning the wedding garment, we

---

8   In the essay "The Weight of Glory" in the book by the same name.
9   The Greek word for sin, ἁμαρτία, comes from the root of ἁμαρτάνω, which means "I miss" (the target).

learn the true significance of what we have done as well as the true significance of what we can become.

We often hear the question, why is the Church so bothered about sex? Yes, the Church does care about sexual immorality, and this is why: because it goes to the heart of what it means to be made in the image of God, to relate to God. Because what we believe and live out physically and temporally in this area of our lives is an icon of a deeper spiritual and eternal reality. And in the light of the full, true meaning of marriage that we have discussed, any way of seeing the world and each other that fails to allow us to see through the veils and takes our eye away from God is pornographic—an obscene writing that obscures rather than reveals the true iconographic nature of created reality.

I do not want to live in this pornographic life of masks. In the end, my deepest desire is to avoid making my life a preparation for a masked ball where nobody is who they seem and all motives are hidden. Rather, I want to accept the veil, don the wedding garment, and attend the wedding supper of the Bridegroom of the Church, where I will in the final consummation truly be seen face to face.

A Prayer of Invitation[10]

I see Thy bridal chamber adorned, O my Savior,
and I have no wedding garment that I may enter there.
Make the robe of my soul to shine, O Giver of Light,
and save me.

---

10 Troparion for Monday, Tuesday, and Wednesday of Holy Week's Bridegroom Services (usually served on the preceding evenings). *Triodion*, 514, 527, 538.

PART 4

Faces

My soul thirsted for the living God: When will I come and appear before the face of God?

—Psalm 41:3 (42:2)

CHAPTER 14

The Beautiful Face of St. Mary of Egypt

THE PROCESS OF RECOGNIZING AND then coming out from behind our masks so that our true faces can be discerned behind the veils of this earthly life is a process of repentance, of turning from a life of *porneia* to a life of the fullness of communion. Each year in church we have an opportunity in our encounter with St. Mary of Egypt to hear how we can live out this process. The life of St. Mary of Egypt, as recorded by St. Sophronius of Jerusalem, is unusual among saints' lives in that it is read in its fullness liturgically, in the Matins of the Great Canon in the fifth week of Great Lent. She is also commemorated on the fifth Sunday of Lent, as well as on her feast day of April 1. Her life story is an icon of repentance, and its contours, I hope, are reflected in the processes and experiences recorded in previous chapters of this book. (See color photo insert F.)

Saint Mary's *Life* reveals how she turns a pornographic life—one focused on the body and on attempts to find fulfillment in physical pleasures and connections—into a life one of the hymns describes as an angelic life while still in the body.[1] The turning point for St. Mary

---

1   Canticle Eight of the second canon on the Thursday of the Great Canon in Lent, *Triodion*, 409.

is an encounter with the icon of the Mother of God—an encounter she describes as beginning when she turns her "bodily and spiritual eyes"[2] on the icon. That is to say, she looks on the icon and sees it as it were with her body and spirit in unity, not her fleshly or masked eyes uninformed by her *nous*. Looking in this way reveals to her the stark contrast between the life she herself has lived up until this point and the life of purity the other Mary, the Most Holy Theotokos, embodies. This leads her to embark on a life of repentance, to accomplish the most remarkable ascetic feats, and to reach such heights of holiness that the purest and holiest of monks, St. Zosimas, on meeting her sees what little he has achieved and how much further from the divine life he is than St. Mary.

I love to hear this story read in church and encourage you to read it again now (you can find it online).[3] But in church in Lent, it comes in the context of the canon of St. Andrew of Crete reflecting on the life of repentance, and juxtaposed with the verses relating to St. Mary herself. This is the best way to hear and prayerfully reflect on it.

As she tells it to St. Zosimas, St. Mary's story begins when she is twelve years old, running away from home in Egypt to its then capital, the international Greek city of Alexandria. There, she launches herself on a life, not even as a prostitute, but as one who gives her body away for nothing (so as not to limit those who want her). She lives off charity and the proceeds of some menial work, but she uses the demand for her sexual services to obtain other things that take her fancy—such as a trip to Jerusalem, which is where she encounters the icon of the Theotokos. Although she offers no excuses or explanations when she tells her story, such behavior would almost certainly be the result of abuse and trauma in childhood.

---

2   Andrew of Crete, *Great Canon*, 88.
3   Current links will usually be found in the "External Links" section of either the OrthodoxWiki or Wikipedia websites' "Mary of Egypt" entry.

In contrast, St. Zosimas came from a monastery in Palestine, where he had been since he was a child. He had grown in learning and holiness, and gained significant renown as an elder and great ascetic. He is described as living a life of repentance and growing so close to perfection that he could no longer find anyone who could teach him. Both St. Zosimas and St. Mary are led to the Jordan: St. Zosimas by a mysterious presence who appears and tells him there is someone there from whom he can learn more about the divine life, and St. Mary by the Mother of God in her icon, to whom St. Mary has promised obedience.

Saint Mary, who was never without companionship, never without physical contact, but somehow was never fulfilled by any of it, ends her life as a hermit, entirely alone in the desert and yet fully in communion with all. Despite (actually, because of) her long desert sojourn, she knows St. Zosimas's name, his history, and all about his brother monks and their monastery rule. Her physical needs are minimal at this point, after astounding feats of fasting and having her flesh thoroughly weathered by years of desert sun and cold nights without clothes, but she has one desire that Fr. Zosimas can fulfill for her. She would like to receive Communion again, as she has lived forty-seven years in the desert without having the opportunity to receive.

Under pressure from St. Zosimas to tell of her experience, St. Mary describes her time in the desert—her own experience of standing "on the verge," as St. Silouan put it—where she was able to keep her mind in hell and yet did not despair. Her story is one of staying in that liminal place where the outcome is unknown, where the desires remain strong and there is no way to meet them. First she experienced the desire for meat and wine, which she had loved so much in Egypt, coupled with the urge to sing the lewd songs of her youth. She brought to her mind the icon of the Theotokos and cried out to her for help. Eventually, she says, light would begin to shine until it covered her, and then peace would descend. But worse were the sexual desires;

like a fire within, she describes them. She would throw herself to the ground and weep for hours on end, but would turn her spiritual eyes to the icon of the Theotokos and ask for help. Here too, in the end, the light would come and she would find herself at peace.

Significantly, these tortures—"wild beasts—mad desires and passions"[4]—lasted for seventeen years, exactly the same amount of time that her pornified life had lasted before she encountered the icon. There was no sudden one-off miraculous cure for her, but the ongoing process of repentance in those seventeen years in the desert—a mirror image of her previous life—was nonetheless miraculous. After these years of suffering had passed, she had experienced another thirty years of living in the desert before St. Zosimas arrived, but she gives us no details about this part of her holy life. Despite this passage of time, when St. Zosimas presses her to tell him about the temptations, she is still reticent, concerned lest bringing them back to mind, she will be tempted again.

This tells us something about the nature of sanctity and the nature of repentance, and also relates to the process of habit and addiction discussed earlier in this book. True repentance is not a momentary change but a mode of living. Although the overcoming of addictions and other issues is often called "recovery," the word *recovery* suggests a return to a way of life previously experienced. For St. Mary of Egypt the sense is that this is more a *dis*covery than a *re*covery—she finds a new path and in repentance turns decisively to follow it. *Healing* in this sense is not the same as *cure*—healing and repentance speak of a path followed, a life lived, not a short-term medication or a surgical procedure. Healing is a process that we are intimately involved in rather than something that is done to us. We may have experiences on that path that are akin to a surgical procedure, but in most cases, they are unlikely to effect a cure on their own.

---

4   Andrew of Crete, *Great Canon*, 90.

Transformation is a real change, but it is not usually instant, and it is also not a magical change into a whole different person. And this is reassuring—love changes me, but I remain myself. Saint Mary the hermit in the desert was in some ways very different from the young Mary the dissolute woman, but she was fully aware of the continuity of her life. She remembered who she was and what she had been, and to go back in her memories even simply in order to tell her story was personally challenging to her. Her past temptation and suffering were still in some sense within her—not just in her mind, but in body, mind, and spirit. In her advanced state of holiness, nothing of her life had been lost. Even in the resurrection, nothing is lost, but those things that were marks of suffering and darkness in this life become glorious in the next—just as the wounds of Christ's suffering on the Cross remain in His resurrection body, but now glorified.

In fact, these marks of suffering and darkness can begin to shine brightly even in this life, as St. Mary's story illustrates. Like a porn user, St. Mary was always looking for love, right from the beginning of her story. She was looking at first in places she could never find it and, like the prodigal son, she came eventually to a realization of that truth of her position—she came to herself[5] and an awareness of how far she was from true love. But she also discovered where the true love was to be found. Once she knew this, she determined to set out on that journey, no matter how difficult. She completed it a full forty-eight years later.

Saint Zosimas, on the other hand, came from a very different place. He had maintained his purity, and yet he was lost. Despite his ascetic achievements, holiness, and the respect of people of faith, he was almost in despair—he had reached the end of his road and could not see where to go next. And then he met St. Mary, and his life was changed forever. This holy man fell in love with the beauty of this

---

5   As Luke 15:17 says of the prodigal son, "when he came to himself..."

woman—this woman who had been used and abused by so many men, who had fasted so that her body was wasted, who had been burned by the sun and frozen at nights so that her flesh was weathered and coarse, and who was already an old woman by the time he met her. What must she have looked like in her youth, when she was desired by so many? And yet, then her true face was hidden deep behind a mask. And what did she look like in her old age, when life had treated her so harshly? But it was that deeper beauty of her old age that was the true beauty. Saint Zosimas saw her face to face, and how could he not love her? When she was young, her fleshly mask, her body of death, was enticing to many. When she was old, those such as St. Zosimas with the eyes to see could perceive her beauty. Her physical body was at this point the thinnest of veils reflecting and revealing the beauty within. This is the beauty of St. Mary that we can also see as we meet her through her icon.

If someone told me they were going to tell me the story of how a sex addict or a prostitute or a porn actress met a holy monk, I don't think this is the story I would expect—that the encounter with the woman would be the monk's salvation. And yet I think it was so.

It is in this way that the marks of what St. Mary describes as her "shame" are also the marks of her holiness and her glory. It is in revealing her true face, in living through her life's experience, that she found holiness, not in hiding it behind a mask. From behind a mask, there is no way forward. Even a mask of holiness will prevent me from finding true holiness; my true face—however dirty and disfigured—is my only hope of discovering it. Likewise, an ersatz holiness is a mask that dulls my eyes and will prevent me from seeing the true face of others. My ways are not God's ways, and what I "know" in terms of my estimation of any other person I would do best to *unknow* if I am to have a hope of seeing the world as God sees it, and of seeing other people the way God sees them. What would I have seen had I met St. Mary in her youth? God saw the saint and called her forth.

Saint Mary reaches such a state of holiness not despite her sin, but through it—by acknowledging and accepting it, facing it, and ultimately transcending it. In her faithful trust and holiness, her fear is cast away, her masks are no longer needed, and her veils are translucent, revealing her true face. She is transformed, and in being transformed becomes more fully and openly herself. She becomes holy through all those years in the desert of refusing to escape from that liminal place, *on the verge*, where her mind is in hell, and yet she does not despair. Saint Zosimas, for all his own holiness, is in awe of her for what she has lived through and what it has led her to become. Saint Mary herself, though, in her humility, seems unaware of this. She constantly defers to St. Zosimas, asking for his blessing, and is always troubled when he asks for hers.

Saint Zosimas brings Communion to St. Mary during the following year's Holy Week, as she has requested. She finishes the prayer for him, and, "according to the custom of that time gave him the kiss of peace on the lips."[6] How many men has she kissed on the lips, and what has it meant to her? There is great significance in the fact that she is enabled, at this point, to give and receive such intimate physical contact in pure love and holiness,[7] and that this is a part of the process of receiving the Body and Blood of Christ, of becoming "one flesh with Him through communion."[8] After receiving, with tears in her eyes, she raises her eyes and hands to heaven and says, "Now lettest Thou Thy servant depart in peace, O Lord, according to Thy word; for my eyes have seen Thy salvation."[9] With these words, as she receives the Body of Christ into her body, she echoes the way Simeon's life

6   Andrew of Crete, *Great Canon*, 94.
7   See Rachel Moran, *Paid For*, part 3, on the challenges for a former prostitute of experiencing loving physical intimacy.
8   Chrysostom, Homily 20 on Ephesians 5:22–33, *On Marriage and Family Life*, 51.
9   Andrew of Crete, 94, based on Luke 2:29–30, part of the usual post-Communion prayers, e.g. *Prayer Book*, 378.

was fulfilled and completed as he received into his arms the infant Christ. Although St. Zosimas did not find it out for another year, St. Mary died that same night and now dwells in the everlasting light, the foretaste of which she received in the desert of her repentance from the icon of the Theotokos.

When I stand in front of the icon of St. Mary of Egypt, tears often come to my eyes as I remember the story of her life. Like St. Zosimas, I have been struck by her beauty, and I wonder what she sees when she looks out at me.

> *The holy Zosimas was struck with amazement, O Mother,*
> *beholding in thee a wonder truly strange and new.*
> *For he saw an angel in the body*
> *and was filled with astonishment,*
> *praising Christ unto all ages.*[10]
> (See color photo insert F.)

---

10   Canticle Eight, Matins Canon on Thursday of the Great Canon, *Triodion*, 409.

CHAPTER 15

Confession: Discovering My True Face

S AINT MARY OF EGYPT'S REPENTANCE began when she came to herself, that is, when she in humility was able to see something of the truth of her life. She described it with the words, "the word of salvation gently touched the eyes of my heart."[1] This is the moment that she began to come out from behind her masks, enabling her to see and be seen. In this moment she began the journey of discovering her true face.

Saint Isaac the Syrian is emphatic about the significance of reaching this point of self-awareness and self-knowledge in truth:

> The man who sighs over his soul for but one hour is greater than he who raises the dead by his prayer. . . . The man who is deemed worthy to see himself is greater than he who is deemed worthy to see the angels, for the latter has communion through his bodily eyes, but the former through the eyes of his soul.[2]

---

1   Andrew of Crete, *Great Canon*, 88.
2   Homily 64, *Ascetical Homilies*, 461.

This process of coming to ourselves, of seeing who we really are, of showing our true faces—this is the process of confession. It is sometimes thought that the English word *confession* has different meanings—including admitting or disclosing guilt and wrongdoing, telling the story of life experience (as, for example, in St. Augustine's *Confessions*), and stating allegiance to a creed (a confession of faith). However, there is really only one meaning here—that of acknowledging Truth, referring to ourselves as icons of Christ, the Logos of God. To confess is to reveal the true face that iconically embodies the hidden nature of a person. The Greek word for confession is ἐξομολόγησις *(exomologesis)*, which could be expressed as showing forth the likeness of the *Logos*, bringing together what is seen or heard outwardly with the true meaning within. This is why Confession precedes Communion: in order to experience a union of love, a full participation in the Body of Christ, we need to be able to see and be seen face to face. Without finding a way to come to know my true face, this is impossible.

So confession is primarily about revealing my true face. This is also what makes forgiveness possible. Without a real acknowledgement of what is wrong, I cannot receive and accept forgiveness, and I cannot take the opportunity for repentance: I need to see that I have fallen in order to get up and try again. Confession is a place for openness and honesty where I can share my deepest fears and anxieties, ask for help with aspects of my life I cannot manage, and receive support to see beyond the masks and veils that obscure who I am in truth. Lifting my masks removes many burdens and refreshes me so that I can find the ongoing path of repentance.

Many of us use some form of structure to prepare for confession, and this can mean that my confession consists of a list of sins I have committed. Looking at my conduct in terms of deeds, words, and thoughts is an important part of self-examination, but it is only the most external part. As I learn to remove my masks and understand the iconological meaning of the veils that cover my true self, rather than just confessing what I have done, I can begin to learn how to confess who I am. That is, I can look down into my heart—into the deep, dark places—and confess the inmost parts of myself, those things that most profoundly inform and underlie my way of life.

It is easy in self-examination to be misled by the image I have of myself (made up of my masks), and I may often get confused between the person I want to be and the person I actually am. This happens when I look at the shiny surface of my soul and think that's all there is. So when I examine myself before confession, I need to go deeper. In the shiny surface of my soul, I see that I want to do good to others, respect them, and see them as the image of God. I can acknowledge that I have not always succeeded, but this seems to be my genuine and full desire. But if I look behind the shiny surface, the mask, if I dig deeper into my heart and my desires, I can find times when my real desire has in fact been to lust after another person—and in so doing, I have abused rather than venerated the image of God in that person.

If my self-examination or introspection goes no further than routinely seeing only the shiny surface, it will distance me further and further from my true face as I fail to suspect what lies beneath the mask. And what lies beneath may be dormant—until suddenly I enter a crisis in my life, which gradually starts to reveal the deeper darkness within. The word *crisis* comes from the Greek for judgment or decision: a crisis will often deliver a decisive judgment about the truth of my masks and will therefore also be a blessing, in that it will help me discern my true face beneath. The Fathers tell us that it is important to know ourselves, but how many of us can really say that we do—really, deep down into the heart?

This is one of the reasons we fast and practice ascetic exercises—in the absence of a crisis, it is a way we begin to gain insight into the truth of who we are beneath the mask. When I am comfortable and life is relatively straightforward, it is easy to look at the shiny surface and believe that this is my true self, whereas in fact it is just a reflection of the blessings of my experience. When I fast, I make life more challenging and the cracks become obvious in the shiny facade of the mask, enabling me to begin to detect my true face beneath.

If we don't know ourselves deeply, as we confess what we have done, we are tempted to see sin more as the breaking of rules than the deforming of persons. And if we think this way about ourselves, it becomes natural to think this way of others as well. I might say, "Why can't he just not do that?" But what if I could see this not just as a rhetorical question, but as a very live one: Why indeed? Why can't *I* just not do that? What is it in the depths of my heart that causes me to react and behave in this particular sinful way? These are the dragons[3] playing beneath the shiny surface of my soul, and just through learning to see them, I will deprive them of much of their power.

Recall the story of the bishops' reactions in Antioch when the scantily clad woman rode by. Those who looked away might have congratulated themselves on their purity. According to the shiny surface of their souls, they were avoiding sin and cultivating purity. And yet it was the holy bishop who did not avert his eyes whose deeper heart was pure. The picture for the others was more complicated—despite desiring purity, some of them may have believed they had attained a higher level of purity than they had, in truth. Perhaps some of them may have felt they had nothing to confess; they had turned away from temptation—and indeed, to turn away was not wrong and may have been the most appropriate response for them. But if they were to confess their real selves, they would need to acknowledge that it was because of the lust in their hearts that they needed to avert their

---

3   See St. Macarius's description of the dragons playing in the heart, quoted in chapter 4 above.

eyes—and also, that any judgment of their brother who did not turn away was misplaced.

Saint Paul says the law was a teacher, guiding people before they had Christ and the Holy Spirit (Gal. 3:10–29; Rom. 7:7–25). Often we crave a simple and specific rule such as the one some of those bishops probably observed: When there is a risk of being provoked[4] to lust, avert your eyes. This may be a good rule to observe. But living just in the law is not enough. Rather, we need to live in the Spirit, as St. Paul says in Galatians 5:18: "But if you are led by the Spirit, you are not under the law." In the Orthodox Church we do not have canon law; we have canons. This is because it is good to observe a rule of life, but it is not good to be in bondage to law. It was good for some of those bishops to avert their eyes. But it would not have been good for St. Nonnus to have done so, because, in the context of his constant prayer, by observing the woman he was led to bless God for the beauty of His creation. Living by the Spirit does not mean that the law is useless or forgotten—rather, it gives a whole new perspective on life and fulfills the law.

So it is with our understanding of confession. We learn to confess by seeing sin as broken rules, and this is a good lesson. But then we need to go deeper into our own persons, because only after fighting through the deep, dark dragons of the heart can we penetrate to the very center of our being, the *nous*, the eye of the soul through which we see God and through which God's light and life stream into us from the inside. And it is through this internal relationship with God that we discover our true face.

Jesus said that it is not what goes into a person that makes a person impure, but what comes out (Mark 7:15). It is not what the eye sees, what the ear hears, not what I touch or taste or smell that defiles me.

---

4   It is also worth noting the concept of "provocative" here. Who was provoking these bishops to sin? It was not the woman, as the holy bishop's response makes clear. It was the dragon within their own hearts.

It is what happens inside me when I receive inwardly what I am given and process it in myself. What do I do with what I receive? What of me do I put into it before I respond? What of God do I allow inside me to change the way I process what I perceive?

I would like to be like that holy bishop. I suspect we would all like to be like that holy bishop. And yet, what is standing between me and that goal? Not God—He is ever-present and filling all things. We only have to turn to Him fully, and He will share everything with us, as the Parable of the Prodigal Son shows us. So if it is not God standing between me and that union with Him that brings purity and love out of me from the inside, it must be something in me. It turns out that being like that holy bishop is something I want with the shiny surface of my soul, but my soul is full of conflicting desires. It is not pure enough to allow this one desire to comprehend and transform all my other, deeper, darker desires, of which I am often hardly aware. Yet I must try to bring those darker things into my awareness so that I can confess them, so that I can confess the whole of me as I truly am. But to bring those things into awareness means to accept them, to accept that they are currently part of me, even though I would rather not admit it.

This is what it means to discover my true face. I would much rather believe my masks, because I have made them to reflect the person I would like to be. But if I deny the darkness within myself, how can I ever have self-knowledge? And without self-knowledge, how can I truly confess? Recognizing and accepting the darkness within me is the beginning of humility, and the more I embody humility, the better I can confess. And without this honesty about myself—the beginnings of humility—how can I love? The purpose of confession is to prepare me for a union of love. In love I need to open myself to the other—to show my true face. How can I do this if I have not even opened myself to me? If I cannot love, I cannot live by either of the two parts of the greatest commandment: to love the Lord with all my heart and soul, and to love my neighbor as myself.

It is in the context of love—the love of God that emerges from my heart through the *nous*, as well as the love I encounter from God and His creation, which approaches me from outside myself—that I will discover my true face. But who is the real me, if it is not the masks I have made—that is, if I am not defined by the sins I have difficulty breaking free from? The *me* I have been used to detecting when I dare to look behind the surface of any of my masks is a me made up largely of my reactions to my own sins and the sins of others—my hurt, loneliness, pain, abandonment, and trauma. But this is not the extent of me. All these things relate to the sinful context of the world and fallen human nature. All of them relate to evil, not to good. All are still masks that cover my true face.

None of these can ultimately be the real me, as we know that the nature of evil is just a twisting of good. Evil has no independent existence. Masks and veils both depend on the reality they cover for their existence to have any meaning at all. So it is with the sinful aspects of my life. They are all broken forms of good—masks or veils over the goodness of God's creation. Underneath each one is a strength, and it is the nature of these strengths that is the eschatological me, the truest and most real version of me, whose face God can always see through the masks and veils of this damaged and sinful earthly existence.

Accepting myself—accepting these deep, dark parts of me—this actually will turn out to be, against all my expectations, a joyful thing, not a depressing one. It is refusing to accept them that is depressing, as it leaves me cut off from the reality of myself, and thereby not only cuts me off from the chance to heal, but also cuts me off from deeper union with every other reality, every other person, and God. Self-acceptance is joyful because it is freeing, because it opens me to be able to truly give and receive love, to find intimacy with others and with God.

Accepting these parts of me does not mean blessing them or pretending they are good; it simply means accepting that they are part of me—embracing them as part of my reality—confessing them to God, and asking Him to enter in and transform me, to renew my heart and my mind in His love. And if I am able to achieve this in myself, this frees me. This way I discover my true face. And by my freedom, I am free to truly love others and to love God. Saint Paul entreats us to do this—to be willing to lose all our images and ideas about ourselves, all of what we think we are:

> Therefore I call upon you, brothers and sisters, through the compassions of God, to present your bodies as a sacrifice—living, holy, pleasing to God—as your reasonable worship, and not to be conformed to this age, but be transformed by the renewal of your nous so that you prove what is the desire of God, the good and pleasing and perfect. (Rom. 12:1–2)

Seeing how far our world is from what is "good and pleasing and perfect," it is easy to fall into hopelessness—whether we ourselves are caught up in addiction to pornography or sexual sin, or whether we just witness the destruction these addictions bring all around us. But hopelessness collapses us in on ourselves rather than drawing us out. Although confession involves looking inside, we do this so that we can meet God there, and this draws us out of ourselves by revealing our true face. In contrast, hopelessness closes us in behind our masks.

We can live in this world as it really is, even in the face of the ugliest parts of it, because we know that behind all the ugliness is the ongoing truth of the constant and consistent offer of a true communion with God that far transcends every taste of communion we can know in this life—a deeper reality in which our cup will truly run over. And we know what we do in order to prepare for Communion: we fast and we confess. This is the beginning of hope, the beginning of repentance, and the beginning of communion. Through this process, in hope, we look toward those things that are unseen but more real, more deeply true than anything we experience with our physical senses alone. We look forward to that experience of truly and fully seeing and being seen face to face.

Confession may take us to the dark places, but these are also places of hope. Through repentance we can find that life of meaning and communion, of joy and of fulfillment. Without repentance, we can only sink further into existential despair. Repentance may begin in the darkest places of despair, in the pigsty, in sackcloth and ashes, but all this is an image of Christ's descent into hell, which turned out to be the beginning of the Resurrection. The icon of the Resurrection is also the icon of the descent into hell. By His descent to the abyss and His destruction of the gates of hell, Christ remains present to us even in our darkest places. Through that presence, He takes our hand, just as He takes Adam's and Eve's in the icon; He tramples the gates that hold us there, freeing us from death, and He opens for us the gates of heaven.

In confession and repentance, nothing is lost, nothing is forgotten, but everything can be transformed. The path is not easy, not direct, not all one way. But the path is always there, and the journey is available to all, because we all bear within ourselves the image of God, and that image is revealed in our own true face. While there is life, there is hope, as that image is never wiped away. While we live and breathe, the animating force is still with us.

We see now through a mirror, obscurely, but then face to face. Now I know in part, but then I will recognize just as I also was recognized. (1 Cor. 13:12)

CHAPTER 16

Communion: Face to Face

IN CONFESSION WE BEGIN TO discover our true faces. This is possible because when we look deep within ourselves, there we encounter God through the nous. The light in our deepest parts is the Light of Christ, the image of God, which remains in every human person while he or she still lives. Each of us is an icon of Christ, who is the perfect human being, the perfect Image of the Father, as we also are exhorted to be: "Therefore you are to be perfect, just as your Father in the heavens is perfect" (Matt. 5:48). We are designed for that fullness, that light, that perfection. And it is when we go to the deepest place inside ourselves, deeper within than the dragons, that we find the nous, the doorway to communion with God, and the source within ourselves of perfect light. This life is given to us for repentance, so that we may be blessed to be the pure in heart who shall see God (Matt. 5:8) and live (Ex. 33:20).

My soul must be saved, and to be saved I must be known. I am always known by God, but I must learn to know myself (in all honesty and humility) so that I can present my soul back to God and to others, because it is through relationships of love that I will find communion and thereby the fullness of healing. Communion works on many levels, and they are not discontinuous—all relationships entered into

194

in truth are iconologically related to the Communion in which we participate in the Liturgy and that ultimate communion of all in eternity. Running away from myself, hiding or covering my true face with a mask, is hiding from the possibility of communion and therefore from the possibility of life in all its fullness forever. Confession and Communion open up the hope of eschatological fulfillment and eternal life, in contrast to the final despair of the hell of self through the parody of communion on offer in this pornographic world.

To hide behind the mask is to make myself alone, and yet, "it is not good for the person to be alone" (Gen. 2:18). We all know this, and we all search for fulfillment in our own lives. Each one of us is truly and fully a *person*, a word that comes from the Greek word πρόσωπον (*prosopon*), which means "face." Saint Sophrony once commented, when receiving a new nun, that monastic clothing is the most personal of all clothing because only the face is visible. The body (veiled) is contextualized by the face. This is the opposite of a pornographic vision, in which the face is contextualized by the body or the body's actions—because the pornographic is not a personal mode of seeing, but an objectifying one. It is a way of avoiding the face of God.

And because each of us is a person—not just an individual—each of us longs to be face to face, truly loving and truly being loved. This is the promise of the gospel, the good news—that we may find that fulfillment in being face to face with God, the ultimate lover, united with Him and with everyone and everything that is and has ever been in Christ for all eternity. Coming into a face-to-face relationship is how we overcome the divisions between us, and it is also the first step to overcoming all the divisions of the cosmos and beginning to participate in that ultimate union of all.

Saint Maximos the Confessor speaks of the divisions of creation[1]—the first one being when God separated created things

---

1   Ambiguum 41, Louth, *Maximus the Confessor*, 156–62.

from the uncreated. Then He separated the created into the noetic world (the world of the nous) and the world that can be sensed. With the third division, God separated the world that can be sensed into heaven and earth; with the fourth, He divided earth into paradise and the world we know, the inhabited world; and with the fifth, He divided those in the world we know into male and female. Our life of repentance on earth is directed toward the union of all these divisions, and it is through that healing that we will find ultimate fulfillment. In this life we may have a foretaste of that ultimate fulfillment in many ways, the most apparent of which is the direct physical communion with God we experience when we take into our own bodies the Body and Blood of Christ. We also experience a taste of the reunion of earth and heaven when we venerate the icon of a saint. These are mystical acts, sacramental acts, and all of life for us can be mystical and sacramental when we experience it in this way.

Equally, a sexual relationship on earth is a union designed to be an icon of that ultimate communion and fulfillment. It is a great mystery, as St. Paul says (Eph. 5:32). It is a union of what is truly diverse in a voluntary communion of persons—a communion so close that they are considered "one body" (Gen. 2:24; Matt. 19:6; 1 Cor. 6:16).

But in our broken world, this mystery is abused, and my pornographic way of seeing greatly tempts me to try to seek fulfillment of that sexual urge toward communion in a false, demonic way that can never yield the true fulfillment I seek. Pornography is one of the most obvious cultural and physical manifestations of noetic and spiritual blindness and sin. It is tempting because, while freely entering into an intimate face-to-face relationship is the path to communion, it is also a path of loving self-sacrifice, and I want to avoid sacrifice, grief, and loss; I want to avoid coming face to face with my fears and insecurities. When I look with my fleshly eyes (the eyes of my body and my mind), I may see in pornography something that I desire, something that seems as if it will satisfy me. But if I am able to look with my spiritual eyes, I will see instead that what I am looking at are symbols of those very losses, fears, and insecurities I am trying to avoid.

When we understand the world iconologically, it is clear that everything is more than it appears—everything is a mask or veil over something deeper. This is why, in pornography, the anonymous body is not usually enough; context is everything. Most people are not aroused by images of nudity in, for example, medical contexts, or in most artistic portrayals of the naked body. But some of those same people are aroused by pornographic portrayals even when they do not involve nudity. This is because pornography is symbolic—it connects with me precisely through my hurt, loneliness, pain, abandonment, and trauma, which are the shadowy things that I spoke of in the preceding chapter that lie just under the thin and brittle shiny surface of my soul. In chapter 4, I talked about the ways in which these shadows are the parts of my story I do not want to see—those stories that, if I cannot tell them or hear them myself, my life will tell another way. And one of these ways is by drawing me into that kind of pornography whose symbolism connects with my particular struggles in a false promise to relieve them. But rather than being at its mercy, I can learn from this if I have the eyes to see iconologically.

I can learn from this because even pornography, in the end, is not primarily about the *facts*, the physical reality; it is about what lies behind—though what lies behind is not truly perceived (as through the veil) but imagined in fantasy (the viewer's own fantasy, reflected back on the mask). Pornography may be made up of misleading signs and symbols, but ultimately even pornography itself cannot escape from the iconological nature of reality or from the call at the heart of creation—a call toward meaning and truth, a call to connect and join together what is separated, an ever-present hint at the path toward communion. Everything in our experience is iconological. To say this is also to say that everything can already give us a taste of the reunion of these divisions, of the day when Christ will be all in all—when everything will be brought fully and finally into union, into a true communion of love, in which personal distinctions remain but all divisions are overcome.

I think this is what St. Augustine was getting at when he wrote his famous passage about seeking love in created things. When he sought ultimate meaning in the things of this world, he was lost. Instead of being a veil through which he perceived God, creation functioned as a mask that formed a barrier between him and God. But once he encountered God, he understood that everything in creation was relative—that all existence related back to that union with God in the light of which his previous visions of lovely things were as blindness, even though those things were in truth recognizable reflections of the same beauty:

> Late have I loved you, beauty so old and so new: late have I loved you. And see, you were within and I was in the external world and sought you there, and in my unlovely state I plunged into those lovely created things which you made. You were with me, and I was not with you. The lovely things kept me far from you, though if they did not have their existence in you, they had no existence at all. You called and cried out loud and shattered my deafness. You were radiant and resplendent, you put to flight my blindness. You were fragrant, and I drew in my breath and now pant after you. I tasted you, and I feel but hunger and thirst for you. You touched me, and I am set on fire to attain the peace which is yours.[2]

It is when we relate to creation precisely as creation and do not imagine it to be in itself ultimate reality that we are able to truly appreciate it for what it really is. This way we truly see its beauty, and

---

2   Augustine, *Confessions*, 201.

through appreciating its beauty, connect through it to the deeper spiritual reality beyond. It is this deeper reality that is the true answer to all our desires, the source of communion, and the only place we can truly find peace.

For a materialist, this world is the ultimate reality: the physical world, the world of facts, the world we can process with our physical senses. But in truth, this is only a small part of reality, the crudest form, we might say. Higher up St. Maximos's hierarchy of division is the division into the noetic world and the world of the body—and, just as we saw when I talked about imagination and fantasy, the body is an icon of the spirit. Whatever happens inwardly manifests in some way outwardly in the body. The purpose of a life of repentance is to bring the two—body and spirit—together into perfect communion through the nous. Our deepest and truest desire, as we have seen, is aimed at fulfilling this communion in the union of all. Our desire is a thirst for infinity, as Staniloae says,[3] and it is because we have a capacity for infinity that the thirst of our passions is of infinite depth—that is, finite creation alone can never satisfy it. We are not infinite by nature but have the possibility of being so through grace—that is, through a communion that leads ultimately to theosis.

Facts are of this world—they do not have meaning outside the fuller truth of the deeper spiritual reality. The world of facts is the world of objectification. If I take facts as the answer in themselves, this is a pornological vision of the world. If I direct my desire only at finite facts, to objectify, my desire will never be satisfied. Our desires will only be satisfied by infinity, which is the world of possibility. We touch this deeper truth through overcoming the slavery of our masks and opening up our true faces in freedom and unknowing, through developing an encounter into a relationship leading to communion.

---

3   Staniloae, *Orthodox Spirituality*, 78–79.

This becomes possible when we exercise our desire through the veil, by veneration.

When our desire is driven by the passions and leads us to objectify, by its nature this objectification is an unwarranted certainty of knowledge that limits both the freedom of the other to become and our own freedom to be open to encounter another in their personal reality. Without this freedom there can be no love, no communion; as Archimandrite Vasileios tells us, the only thing in the end "that exists outside freedom is hell and death."[4] Objectification, then, is an anti-communion, which ultimately results in the hell of isolation. Objectifying knowledge—the acceptance of a person or thing in creation as just a fact—precludes openness to the other. What we know by senses and cognition alone is only the nonexistent, according to St. Gregory of Nyssa,[5] because by making them facts in their own right, we have separated them (and ourselves) from God—the source of all, the fullness of truth, and the only non-dependent reality.

Objectifying the other is related to the passions, which are essentially acquisitive or appetitive. They are about possessing the other or incorporating what I feel I need or want into myself, rather than encountering the other as a person and being open to connection and communion. Although being seen is what I most yearn for, if I am afraid of the content of my heart and life, I want at least selectively to remain hidden. I want to control what others see. I want to control what I see of myself. Thus, the passions cut off the possibility of fulfilling the very desires in which they are manifest. Objectifying the other ultimately leads to the hell of isolation in the self, where I no longer have the ability to relate. This was illustrated to St. Macarius in a vision in which a spirit in hell told him, "It is not possible to see anyone face to face, but the face of one is fixed to the back of another."

---

4   Vasileios, *Hymn of Entry*, 49.
5   As quoted in Vasileios, 38.

However, he went on, "Yet when you pray for us, each of us can see the other's face a little. Such is our respite."[6] It is through prayer, through the sacramental life, through the mysteries of the Church, that we move from the hell of objectification to veneration and a communion of love. Icons are full-face, and we encounter them face to face. In icons, it is only the demons and the lost who are in profile, not seeing or being seen face to face.

This movement—out of the hell of separation and objectification and into veneration and the ability to see and be seen face to face in a communion of love—is exactly what we see and do when we participate in the Divine Liturgy. There we gather as the Church, leave behind all earthly cares and the fleshly nature of this world, and approach Communion. This Communion we approach in the Liturgy connects with the deeper reality of each and all, integrating the whole world and all relationships mystically into communion, overcoming every division. In the Divine Liturgy we participate in the move from an objectified life of fact to a life of participation in the reality beyond the senses and the reality of each other. In the Liturgy we complete the action we began in confession, of removing our masks of death and exposing our true faces to a life-giving face-to-face encounter. In the Liturgy we move from death to life—from crucifixion to resurrection. In the Liturgy, just as in the icon, we experience that radical transformation of perspective: proportions and sizes all seem different; the distances of time and space are overcome. In the Liturgy, what is divided and distributed unites us as one body: our divisions are transcended, and our personhood is fulfilled as we are joined in communion. As Archimandrite Vasileios says, "In the Divine Liturgy, things are different: we learn to love."[7] In the Liturgy, we unite

---

6   Macarius the Great, 38, in Ward, *Sayings of the Desert Fathers*, 156–57.
7   Vasileios, 75.

ourselves to the whole world—visible and invisible. In the Liturgy, nothing is objectified. In the Liturgy, we learn to venerate.

What we have called the iconological way of seeing is a way of seeing that involves veneration. It is the way of seeing that is appropriate to the union of the Logos with the physical, which is possible because of the Incarnation. And it is the Incarnation that makes communion possible—through it, we in the physical world can, as whole persons, body, mind, and spirit, find communion with the divine. The miracle of the Incarnation made possible what had always been impossible— that a human being could see the face of God and yet live. The Incarnation also made the appearance of the holy icons not only justifiable, not only inevitable, but necessary: the safeguard of the faith. Having seen God in the flesh, who would not depict Him? As long as we continue to venerate His image, we cannot deny the reality of the Incarnation.

The Incarnation also makes miracle-working icons inevitable. The union of Logos and the material world means that the whole material world is filled with the potentiality to manifest and find communion with the divine life. Every icon is miracle-working in that it brings into our fallen world an experience of that fuller, perfected life in which the saints dwell. Every miracle is, after all, simply an appearance in this fallen world of the way things ought to be and are in eternity. Our encounter with the divine life shining through this earthly existence calls us to venerate, and venerating implies unknowing, purification, and relationship. Just as objectifying is related to a fixed knowledge, venerating implies openness to the dynamic nature of life in relationship, openness to the other in unknowing. In the Liturgy, in order to participate in Communion, we unknow the facts of bread and wine in order to partake of the Holy Body and Blood. In unknowing, we perceive rather than prejudge; we do not limit the possibilities of God, but participate in His energies.

Venerating requires the purification of our eyes so that our bodily eyes can be joined not only with our mind's eye but also with our spiritual eyes. To know this is to know the futility of fighting the evil of pornography—or indeed, any evil—simply, or even mostly, in the physical realm. The search for purity must go much deeper. Purification is the beginning, but through communion, our purification becomes illumination, and then, rather than being drawn to reflect the darkness of a pornified world, our eyes will rather reflect the light of truth, as St. Ephrem the Syrian says:[8]

When it is associated with a source of light
an eye becomes clear:
it shines with the light that provisions it,
it gleams with its brightness,
it becomes glorious with its splendor,
adorned by its beauty.

As we purify our eyes, we find that the way we look at others changes, and this changes them as well as ourselves. When we truly look on others with veneration, their souls will know it, because the act of looking at each other face to face in veneration is itself an iconic action—it symbolizes iconologically the potential fullness of relationship. It is both a recognition of the real potential for a fullness of communion and also an invitation to move toward that fullness; it emerges from a relationship and is part of the process by which that relationship grows and flourishes in an ongoing dynamic process. The look of veneration is, to reuse St. Augustine's phrase in the fuller context, "plunging into" communion.

St. Augustine described himself plunging into created things without an awareness of what he was doing. Plunging into these lovely created things is in truth what we are here to do—but not apart from the

---

8   Hymns on the Church 36.1, Brock, *Bride of Light*, 28. The context of the rest of the hymn adds that the eye of the soul of the Theotokos is enlightened by the light that is Christ received into her womb.

iconological awareness of their true meaning. To plunge in and see the physical things superficially and not iconologically is to see the image and miss the meaning, which is what makes the veil a mask. In veneration, by contrast, we connect with the meaning: we meet the eternal through the physical. We do not confuse the physical with the eternal, but as we are embodied beings, we can only encounter the eternal as whole persons when body, mind, and spirit work together as one. It is in this way we find that God's creation is, indeed, good (Gen. 1). We are washed with the water of baptism to be born again. We kiss the icon to venerate the person of the saint. We eat the Body and drink the Blood of Christ to find union with Him in eternity. We connect in spirit through our actions with the body. This is because God grants all creation by grace the opportunity to participate in that unity which God the Trinity has by nature.

And yet plunging into this communion is a risky and dangerous business. If I answer the invitation to communion, I can never be truly ready, never truly worthy of what I am stepping into: it is so much more than I have dreamed of in my petty passions. When I receive the Body of Christ, I receive a "burning coal."[9] I partake of fire while being made of grass, and yet, like the burning bush that Moses saw, I am not burned up,[10] but rather through receiving this fire, my masks (my sins) can be burned away.[11] Moreover, as in the Cherubic Hymn we stand and offer what we have to be incorporated into this communion, we identify ourselves with the cherubim—the ones who attend God amidst flames of fire (Ezek. 10:6–7). As Abba Lot discovered, when we are fully integrated into this communion of love, we can also reflect the burning light and warmth of His countenance and

---

9   The third prayer of preparation (St. John Chrysostom), Lash, *Orthodox Prayer Book*, 46.
10   The seventh prayer of preparation (St. Symeon the New Theologian), Lash, 51.
11   The verses and troparia following the twelve prayers of preparation, Lash, 54–55.

become "all flame." Abba Lot had asked Abba Joseph what lay beyond his daily practice:

> "Abba, as far as I can I say my little office, I fast a little, I pray and meditate, I live in peace and as far as I can, I purify my thoughts. What else can I do?" Then the old man stood up and stretched his hands towards heaven. His fingers became like ten lamps of fire and he said to him, "if you will, you can become all flame."[12]

Our life is a preparation to be joined in a perfect communion of all in the presence of the face of God. With the cherubim we will then reflect the fire of His love without being burned up in His glory.

We may feel that we are very far from the ability to be "all flame"— very far from readiness to stand with all the saints and the cherubim in the presence of God, face to face. As bearers of His image, we are still far from His likeness. And yet, we have seen that even our struggles are icons of this glory. We all have many gifts to thank God for and to offer to others, and in the end we can see that our superficial desires and addictions are both gift and vocation. Our weaknesses turn out to be themselves gifts, because it is only through death that we can find resurrection—only through our weaknesses that we are made strong. With St. Paul, we hear the Lord say to us, "My grace is enough for you. For My power is perfected in weakness." And St. Paul also tells us, "For this reason I take delight in weaknesses, in insults, in constraints, in persecutions, in distresses, for Christ. For when I am weak, then I am strong" (2 Cor. 12:9–10).

Having prepared ourselves by passing through the death of the mask, of our pornified self-constructions, of our striving to lose ourselves in self-destructive attempts at physical union that block us from true communion, ultimately, we find that we can enter into a

---

12   Joseph of Panephysis, 7, in Ward, *Sayings of the Desert Fathers*, 103.

fuller union than we could ever have imagined. We can step into the fire of love and beauty and become one with it, and reflect all its fullness in our redeemed selves.

As I prepare for communion in this life, then, let my prayer be the kiss of veneration, which is always chaste, as was the kiss of peace St. Mary of Egypt gave to St. Zosimas before she received the Body and Blood. Even if I fear that the pollution is so deep in me that when I kiss the icon, this kiss may not be pure, it does not matter, because Christ, the Mother of God, and the saints are all unimaginably stronger than any of my impurities. So let me kiss the icon with my whole being, without fear, without holding anything back, knowing that nothing in me puts me beyond the love of Christ. In this, I can accept God's love for me as I am—I do not need to be perfect to be truly loved. And equally, being loved in my imperfections does not make my imperfections good; it simply recognizes that they are facts to be transformed into truth. Knowing that God loves me also means knowing not only that it is possible for me to be loved, but that it is good to love me, because God never does anything other than good. I do not need to search after love; I already have it.

As we stand in front of the icon in this way, seeing and being seen face to face, time becomes relative. The moment in front of the icon manifests to us the truth that each present moment is not a fragment of time passing away but a fragment of eternity.

To stand in front of the icon is to stand on the threshold of eternity, on the threshold of communion, and to be seen in truth for everything we are in all the uniqueness and fullness of our personhood. This uniqueness is the reason that, although we are all engaged in a life of repentance, there is not one obvious path common to all. God offers many things, and we must seek out how to respond—not by killing desire, but by finding what God offers that moves our own desire, and then struggling onto that path, holding that ultimate desire resolutely in our hearts, moving toward it by ascetic struggle. Getting up when we fall, without the pride of self-judgment or self-condemnation. I expect to fall because I am weak and sinful. It is through my weakness that I know God's strength. In that strength will I rise and continue.

The path we must follow is not straight, but it is narrow (the common saying comes from a misunderstanding of the Middle English *strait*, meaning "constricted"). There are many twists and turns to negotiate. But we can see our way along the narrow path because our way is lit by Christ, "the joyful Light of the holy glory, of the immortal, heavenly, holy, blessed Father."[13] Christ is the true Light we sing of in the Liturgy and the true Faith we have found. And we see all these things when we meet Him face to face. God never compels us to see Him, but He always and forever offers the vision. We seek Him through a life of continually turning to Him in repentance, by which we purify our vision and grow in love until we are ready to come before His face.

The discovery of our true faces through a life of repentance leading to communion turns out to be, as I said earlier, a joyful thing. "Let no one weep for his transgressions, for forgiveness hath dawned from the tomb,"[14] as St. John Chrysostom reminds us every Pascha. The Paschal fullness is the life we are called to live. Through death in all its forms, we are offered in love that union with the fullness of life and the fullness of beauty that is far beyond any beauty we ever desired with our pornified eyes.

Jesus said, "The one who sees Me has seen the Father" (John 14:9). (See color photo insert G.) To look on Christ with the eye of the heart and in the power of the Holy Spirit is not only to see the Incarnate Son, but to see the invisible Father (Col. 1:15). Christ's humanity is the image of His divinity, and through His assumption of everything

---

13   The hymn *Phos Hilaron* from Vespers.
14   Paschal Homily of St. John Chrysostom.

in our human nature, He shines forth a vision of the perfect likeness. When we unite ourselves with this vision, the glory of the image of God that is in all of us can become in each one of us a perfect likeness of God. And yet, it will be a perfect likeness that also reflects most fully what it means to be distinctly ourselves as we join the communion of all things in love.

Knowing that the seraphim veil their faces as they enter the presence of God's countenance, we even in this earthly life are able to stand and look directly into the face of Christ fully, if we dare. Face to face with Christ, we find all our pornographic desires fall away, as everything of this life is relativized in the light of life eternal. Once our spiritual cataracts have been removed, once the scales fall from our eyes (Acts 9:18), we will find it is not possible to see and love God and also to hate, use, or abuse any other person—physically, mentally, or spiritually, either directly or through an image. When our eyes are finally clear, the masks will no longer obscure, and we will be able to see each hidden person we encounter face to face.

O Bridegroom, surpassing all in beauty, Thou hast called us to the spiritual feast of Thy bridal chamber. Strip from me the disfigurement of sin through participation in Thy sufferings; clothe me in the glorious robe of Thy beauty, and in Thy compassion make me feast with joy at Thy Kingdom.[15]

---

15   From the Aposticha at the Matins of Holy Tuesday, *Triodion*, 528.

References

Articles, Reports, and Websites

Adams, Don. "Can Pornography Cause Rape?" *Journal of Social Philosophy* 31, no. 1 (Spring 2000): 1–43.

Anonymous. "Ask a semi-retired porn star anything." Chan Archive, accessed April 20, 2011. http://chanarchive.org/4chan/b/9395/ask-a-semi-retired -pornstar-anything#323234995. (page inactive)

Attorney General's Commission on Pornography. *Final Report.* Washington, DC: Government Printing Office, 1986.

Barron, Martin, and Michael Kimmel. "Sexual Violence in Three Pornographic Media: Toward a Sociological Explanation." *The Journal of Sex Research* 37, no. 2 (May 2000): 161–168.

British Board of Film Classification (BBFC). *Young people, Pornography and Age-verification* (London: British Board of Film Classification: 2020).

Begovic, Hamdija. "Pornography Induced Erectile Dysfunction Among Young Men." *Dignity: A Journal of Analysis of Exploitation and Violence* 4, no. 1 (2019): Article 5.

Blair, Linsey. "How difficult is it to treat delayed ejaculation within a short-term psychosexual model? A case study comparison." *Sexual and Relationship Therapy* 33, no. 3 (2018): 298–308.

Bőthe, Beáta, István Tóthe-Király, Nóra Bella, Marc N. Potenza, Zsolt Demetrovics, and Gábor Orosz. "Why do people watch pornography? The motivational basis of pornography use." *Psychology of Addictive Behaviors* 35, no. 2 (March 2021): 172–186.

Bridges, Ana, Robert Wosnitzer, Erica Scharrer, Chyng Sun, and Rachael Liberman. "Aggression and Sexual Behavior in Best-Selling Pornography Videos: A Content Analysis Update." *Violence Against Women* 16, no. 10 (2010): 1065–1085.

Coleman, John. "Porn in the USA." *Salvo* 2, Spring 2007. https://salvomag.com/article/salvo2/porn-in-the-usa.

Donevan, Meghan. "'In This Industry, You're No Longer Human': An Exploratory Study of Women's Experiences in Pornography Production in Sweden." *Dignity: A Journal of Analysis of Exploitation and Violence* 6, no. 3 (2021): Article 1.

Esplin, Charlotte, S. Gabe Hatch, H. Dorian Hatch, Conner L. Deichman, and Scott R. Braithwaite. "What motives drive pornography use?" *The Family Journal* 29, no. 2 (2021): 161–174.

Flood, Michael, and Clive Hamilton. "Youth and Pornography in Australia: evidence on the extent of exposure and likely effects." Discussion Paper No. 52, The Australia Institute, 2003.

Flood, Michael. "Pornography, violence and popular debate." *DVRCV Advocate*, Spring/Summer 2013, 42–44.

Gavrieli, Ran. "Pornografie Ist Gefilmte Prostitution!" *Emma*, December 12, 2013. https://www.emma.de/artikel/pornografie-ist-gefilmte-prostitution-312969.

HM Government. *Working Together to Safeguard Children: A guide to inter-agency working to safeguard and promote the welfare of children.* London: HM Government, 2018. https://www.gov.uk/government/publications/working-together-to-safeguard-children--2.

Green, Bradley A., Stefanie Carnes, Patrick J. Carnes, and Elizabeth A. Weinman. "Cybersex Addiction Patterns in a Clinical Sample of Homosexual, Heterosexual, and Bisexual Men and Women." *Sexual Addiction & Compulsivity* 19, no. 1–2 (2012): 77–98.

Grudzen, Corita R., Gery Ryan, William Margold, Jacqueline Torres, and Lillian Gelberg. "Pathways to Health Risk Exposure in Adult Film Performers." *Journal of Urban Health* 86, no. 1 (January 2009): 67–78.

Grudzen, Corita, Daniella Meeker, Jacqueline Torres, Qingling Du, R. Sean Morrison, Ronald M. Andersen, and Lillian Gelberg. "Comparison of the Mental Health of Female Adult Film Performers and Other Young Women in California." *Psychiatric Services* 62, no. 6 (June 2011): 639–645.

Harpaz, Beth J. "Hyatt hotels banning on-demand porn movies in hotel rooms." *AP News*, October 14, 2015. https://apnews.com/article/769fcab3b9134307b05beffd423d7da5.

References

Henry, Nicola, and Alice Witt. "Governing Image-Based Sexual Abuse: Digital Platform Policies, Tools, and Practices." In *The Emerald International Handbook of Technology Facilitated Violence and Abuse,* edited by Jane Bailey, Asher Flynn, and Nicola Henry, 749–768. Bingley, England: Emerald Publishing, 2021.

Javanbakht, Marjan, M. Claire Dillavou, Robert W. Rigg, Peter R. Kerndt, and Pamina M. Gorbach. "Transmission Behaviors and Prevalence of Chlamydia and Gonorrhea Among Adult Film Performers." *Sexually Transmitted Diseases* 44, no. 3 (March 2017): 181–186.

Khalili. "These are the most popular websites in the world—And they might just surprise you." *TechRadar,* 2021 on https://www.techradar.com/news/porn -sites-attract-more-visitors-than-netflix-and-amazon-youll-never-guess -how-many. Accessed August 20, 2019. (page inactive)

Lambert, Nathaniel M., Sesen Negash, Tyler F. Stillman, Spencer B. Olmstead, and Frank D. Fincham. "A love that doesn't last: Pornography consumption and weakened commitment to one's romantic partner." *Journal of Social and Clinical Psychology* 31, no. 4 (2012): 410–438.

Lim, Megan S. C., Paul A. Agius, Elise R. Carrotte, Alyce M. Vella, and Margaret E. Hellard. "Young Australians' use of pornography and associations with sexual risk behaviours." *Australia and New Zealand Journal of Public Health* 41, no. 4 (August 2017): 438–443.

Malamuth, Neil. "Pornography." In *International Encyclopedia of Social and Behavioral Sciences,* Vol. 17, edited by N. J. Smelser and P. B. Baltes, 11816–11821. (Amsterdam: Elsevier, 2001).

Marshall, Ethan A., Holly A. Miller, and Jeffrey A. Bouffard. "Bridging the Theoretical Gap: Using Sexual Script Theory to Explain the Relationship Between Pornography Use and Sexual Coercion." *Journal of Interpersonal Violence* 36, no. 9–10 (May 2021): NP5215–NP5238.

Mirzaei, Yaser, Somayyeh Zare, and Todd G. Morrison. "Hijab Pornography: A Content Analysis of Internet Pornographic Videos." *Violence Against Women* 28, no. 6–7 (2022): 1420–1440.

Mohan, Megha. "'I was raped at 14, and the video ended up on a porn site'." *BBC,* February 10, 2020. https://www.bbc.co.uk/news/stories-51391981.

Negash, Sesen, Nicole Van Ness Sheppard, Nathaniel M. Lambert, and Frank D. Fincham. "Trading Later Rewards for Current Pleasure: Pornography Consumption and Delay Discounting." *Journal of Sex Research* 53, no. 6 (July–August 2016): 689–700.

Martellozzo, Elena, Andrew Monaghan, Joanna Adler, Rodolfo Leyva, Julia Davidson, and Miranda Horvath. *"I wasn't sure it was normal to watch it . . .": A quantitative and qualitative examination of the impact of online pornography on the values, attitudes, beliefs and behaviours of children and young people.* (London: Middlesex University, NSPCC, Children's Commissioner, 2016).

"Non-consensual nudity policy." Twitter, December, 2021. https://help.twitter .com/en/rules-and-policies/intimate-media.

Park, Brian Y., Gary Wilson, Jonathan Berger, Matthew Christman, Bryn Reina, Frank Bishop, Warren P. Klam, and Andrew P. Doan. "Is Internet Pornography Causing Sexual Dysfunctions? A Review with Clinical Reports." *Behavioral Sciences* 6, no. 3 (September 2016): 17.

Pennsylvania Department of Corrections. *Correctional Newsfront,* 2006, 32–33.

Porto, R. "Habitudes masturbatoires et dysfonctions sexuelles masculines." *Sexologies* 25, no. 4 (August 2016): 160–165.

Puddephatt, Andrew. "Pornhub: Data out of context tells us nothing." Internet Watch Foundation, December 15, 2020. https://www.iwf.org.uk/news /pornhub-data-out-of-context-tells-us-nothing.

Rimm, Martin. "Marketing Pornography on the Information Superhighway: A Survey of 917,410 Images, Description, Short Stories and Animations Downloaded 8.5 Million Times by Consumers in Over 2000 Cities in Forty Countries, Provinces and Territories." *Georgetown Law Journal* 83, no. 5 (1996): 1849–1934.

Tyler, Meagan. "Harms of production: theorising pornography as a form of prostitution." *Women's Studies International Forum* 48 (Jan–Feb 2015): 114–123.

U.S. Attorney's Office, Southern District of California. "GirlsDoPorn Employee Pleads Guilty to Sex Trafficking Conspiracy," April 16, 2021. https:// www.justice.gov/usao-sdca/pr/girlsdoporn-employee-pleads-guilty-sex -trafficking-conspiracy.

Vera-Gray, Fiona, Clare McGlynn, Ibad Kureshi, and Kate Butterby. "Sexual violence as a sexual script in mainstream online pornography." *The British Journal of Criminology* 61, no. 5 (September 2021): 1–18.

Wéry, Aline, Natale Canale, Caroline Bell, Benoit Duvivier, and Joël Billieux. "Problematic online sexual activities in men: The role of self-esteem, loneliness, and social anxiety." *Human Behavior and Emerging Technologies* 2, no. 3 (2020): 217–226.

Wright, Paul J., Debby Herbenick, Bryant Paul, and Robert S. Tokunaga. "Exploratory Findings on U.S. Adolescents' Pornography Use, Dominant Behavior, and Sexual Satisfaction." *International Journal of Sexual Health* 33, no. 2 (2021): 222–228.

Books

Aggeloglou, Christodoulos. *Elder Paisios of the Holy Mountain*. Mount Athos, Greece: Holy Mountain, 1998.

Alcoholics Anonymous. *Alcoholics Anonymous: The Story of How Many Thousands of Men and Women Have Recovered from Alcoholism*. New York: Alcoholics Anonymous World Services, 2001.

Andrew of Crete. *The Great Canon: The Work of St. Andrew of Crete*. Translated by Kallistos Ware and Holy Trinity Monastery. Jordanville, NY: Holy Trinity Publications, 2016.

Arendt, Hannah. *Eichmann in Jerusalem: A Report on the Banality of Evil*. London: Penguin, 2006.

———. *Love and Saint Augustine*. Translated and edited by Joanna Vecchiarelli Scott and Judith Chelius Stark. Chicago: University of Chicago Press, 1996.

Athanasius. *On the Incarnation*. Translated and edited by a Religious of CSMV. Crestwood, NY: St. Vladimir's Seminary Press, 1982.

Augustine. *Confessions*. Translated and edited by Henry Chadwick. Oxford: Oxford University Press, 2008.

Beausobre, Iulia de. *Creative Suffering*. Oxford: SLG Press, 1984.

———. *The Woman Who Could Not Die*. London: Chatto and Windus, 1938.

Book of Akathists. Jordanville, NY: Holy Trinity Monastery, 1994.

Book of Hours, The. Boston: Holy Transfiguration Monastery, 2014.

Boss, Sarah Jane. *Empress and Handmaid: On Nature and Gender in the Cult of the Virgin Mary*. London: Cassell, 2000.

Boyle, Karen, ed. *Everyday Pornography*. Abingdon, UK: Routledge, 2010.

Breck, John. *The Sacred Gift of Life: Orthodox Christianity and Bioethics*. Crestwood, NY: St. Vladimir's Seminary Press, 1998.

Brock, Sebastian. *Bride of Light: Hymns on Mary from the Syriac Churches*. Kerala, India: St. Ephrem Ecumenical Research Institute, 1994.

Brown, Brené. *Daring Greatly: How the Courage to Be Vulnerable Transforms the Way We Live, Love, Parent, and Lead*. London: Penguin, 2013.

Chrysostom, John. *On Marriage and Family Life*. Translated by Catherine P. Roth and David Anderson. Crestwood, NY: St. Vladimir's Seminary Press, 2003.

Climacus, John. *The Ladder of Divine Ascent*. Boston: Holy Transfiguration Monastery, 2001.

Cox, John, Alastair V. Campbell, and Bill Fulford. *Medicine of the Person: Faith, Science and Values in Health Care Provision*. London: Jessica Kingsley, 2007.

Doidge, Norman. *The Brain That Changes Itself: Stories of Personal Triumph from the Frontiers of Brain Science.* London: Penguin, 2007.

Dzalto, Davor. *The Human Work of Art: A Theological Appraisal of Creativity and the Death of the Artist.* Yonkers, NY: St. Vladimir's Seminary Press, 2014.

Evdokimov, Paul. *The Art of the Icon: A Theology of Beauty.* Redondo Beach, CA: Oakwood Publications, 1990.

Foucault, Michel. *The History of Sexuality, Volume 1: An Introduction.* Translated by Robert Hurley. New York: Vintage Books, 1990.

Florensky, Pavel. *Iconostasis.* Translated by Donald Sheehan and Olga Andrejev. Crestwood, NY: St. Vladimir's Seminary Press, 1996.

Gregory the Great. *Forty Gospel Homilies.* Translated by David Hurst. Trappist, KY: Cistercian Publications, 1990.

Gregory of Nyssa. *The Lord's Prayer. The Beatitudes.* Translated and edited by Hilda C. Graef. Mahwah, NJ: Paulist Press, 1954.

Hari, Johann. *Chasing the Scream: The First and Last Days of the War on Drugs.* London: Bloomsbury, 2015.

Hierotheos, Metropolitan of Nafpaktos. *Orthodox Psychotherapy: The Science of the Fathers.* Translated by Esther Williams. Levadia, Greece: Birth of the Theotokos Monastery, 1994.

Hügel, Friedrich von. *Essays and Addresses on the Philosophy of Religion: Second Series.* London: J. M. Dent & Sons, 1926.

Isaac the Syrian. *The Ascetical Homilies of St. Isaac the Syrian.* Boston: Holy Transfiguration Monastery, 1984.

John of Damascus. *Three Treatises on the Divine Images.* Translated by Andrew Louth. Crestwood, NY: St. Vladimir's Seminary Press, 2003.

John of Kronstadt. *My Life in Christ.* Translated by E. E. Goulaeff. Jordanville, NY: Holy Trinity Publications, 1977.

Johnson, Samuel. *The Rambler.* In Three Volumes. Volume the Second. The Sixteenth Edition. London: n. p., 1806.

Lash, Ephrem, trans. and ed. *An Orthodox Prayer Book.* Oxford: Oxford University Press, 1999.

Lewis, C. S. *The Collected Letters of C. S. Lewis, Volume 3: Narnia, Cambridge, and Joy, 1950–1963.* London: HarperCollins, 2004.

———. *The Great Divorce, A Dream.* London: G. Bles, 1945.

———. *The Weight of Glory.* New York: HarperCollins, 2001.

Lossky, Vladimir. *The Mystical Theology of the Eastern Church.* Translated by the Fellowship of St. Alban and St. Sergius. Crestwood, NY: St. Vladimir's Seminary Press, 1976.

References

Louth, Andrew. *Maximus the Confessor.* London: Routledge, 1996.

MacKinnon, Catharine A., and Andrea Dworkin, eds. *In Harm's Way: The Pornography Civil Rights Hearings.* Cambridge, MA: Harvard University Press, 1997.

Manoussakis, John Panteleimon. *God after Metaphysics: A Theological Aesthetic.* Bloomington, IN: Indiana University Press, 2007.

Manual of Eastern Orthodox Prayers, A. London: SPCK, 1945.

Marion, Jean-Luc. *The Crossing of the Visible.* Translated by James K. A. Smith. Redwood City, CA: Stanford University Press, 2004.

Mary, Mother and Kallistos Ware, trans. and eds. *The Lenten Triodion.* London: Faber & Faber, 1978.

Mason, A. J. *Fifty Spiritual Homilies of St. Macarius the Egyptian.* London: Society for Promoting Christian Knowledge, 1921.

Maté, Gabor. *In the Realm of Hungry Ghosts: Close Encounters with Addiction.* London: Penguin, 2018.

Mikkola, Mari. *Pornography: A Philosophical Introduction.* New York: Oxford University Press, 2019.

Moran, Rachel. *Paid for: My Journey Through Prostitution.* Dublin: Gill & Macmillan, 2013.

NPNF-I—see Schaff; NPNF-II—see Schaff and Wace.

Norris, Richard A., trans. and ed. *Gregory of Nyssa: Homilies on the Song of Songs.* Atlanta: Society of Biblical Literature, 2012.

Old Orthodox Prayer Book. 3rd ed. Erie, PA: Russian Orthodox Church of the Nativity of Christ, 2015.

Paul, Pamela. *Pornified: How the Culture of Pornography Is Transforming Our Lives, Our Relationships, and Our Families.* New York: Times Books, 2005.

Palmer, G.E.H., Philip Sherrard, and Kallistos Ware, trans. *The Philokalia: The Complete Text.* Vols. 1, 4. London: Faber & Faber, 1983, 1998.

Philokalia—see Palmer.

Powell, Mark E. "Pneumatology and the Canonical Heritage." In *T&T Handbook of Pneumatology,* ed. Daniel Castelo and Kenneth M. Loyer, 337–344. London: Bloomsbury, 2020.

Prayer Book for Orthodox Christians, A. Boston: Holy Transfiguration Monastery, 2014.

Rieber, Robert W., and Harold J. Vetter. *The Psychopathology of Language and Cognition.* New York: Springer, 2013.

Sahas, Daniel J. *Icon and Logos: Sources in Eighth-Century Iconoclasm.* Toronto: University of Toronto Press, 1986.

Schaff, Philip, ed. *Nicene and Post-Nicene Fathers Series I*. Peabody, MA: Hendrickson, 2004. Reprint of the original American edition of 1888.

Schaff, Philip, and Henry Wace, eds. *Nicene and Post-Nicene Fathers Series II*. Peabody, MA: Hendrickson, 2004. Reprint of the original American edition of 1900.

Sophrony (Sakharov), Archimandrite. *Saint Silouan the Athonite*. Translated by Rosemary Edmonds. Maldon, UK: The Patriarchal Stavropegic Monastery of Saint John the Baptist, 1991.

Staniloae, Dumitru. *Orthodox Spirituality: A Practical Guide for the Faithful and a Definitive Manual for the Scholar*. Translated by Jerome Newville and Otilia Kloos. South Canaan, PA: St. Tikhon's Orthodox Theological Seminary Press, 2002.

Tarrant, Shira. *The Pornography Industry: What Everyone Needs to Know*. New York: Oxford University Press, 2016.

Thekla, Abbess, and Mother Katherine. *The Great Canon of St. Andrew of Crete and the Life of Saint Mary of Egypt*. n. p.: Finnan Books, 2013.

Theophan the Recluse. *Unseen Warfare*. Translated by E. Kadloubovsky and G. E. H. Palmer. Crestwood, NY: St. Vladimir's Seminary Press, 1987.

Tolstoy, Leo. *The Death of Ivan Ilyich, the Cossacks, Happy Ever After*. Translated by Rosemary Edmonds. London: Penguin Books, 1960.

Traherne, Thomas. *Centuries of Meditations*. New York: Cosimo Classics, 2010.

Triodion—see Mary, Mother, and Archimandrite Kallistos Ware.

Vasileios, Archimandrite. *Hymn of Entry*. Translated by Elizabeth Briere. Crestwood, NY: St. Vladimir's Seminary Press, 1984.

Velimirovich, Nikolai. *Prayers by the Lake*. Translated and edited by Todor Mika and Stevan Scott. Grayslake, IL: The Serbian Orthodox Metropolitanate of New Gračanica, 1999.

———. *Missionary Letters of Saint Nikolai Velimirovich, Part I*. Translated by Serafim Baltic and edited by Milorad Loncar. Grayslake, IL: New Gračanica Monastery, 2008.

Ward, Benedicta. *Harlots of the Desert: A Study of Repentance in Early Monastic Sources*. Oxford: Mowbray, 1987.

———. *The Sayings of the Desert Fathers: The Alphabetical Collection*. Trappist, KY: Cistercian Publications, 1984.

Weil, Simone. *Gravity and Grace*. Translated by Emma Crawford and Mario von der Ruhr. Abingdon, UK: Routledge, 2002.

Winnicott, D. W. *The Maturational Processes and the Facilitating Environment: Studies in the Theory of Emotional Development*. London: The Hogarth Press and the Institute of Psycho-Analysis, 1965.

Wilson, Gary. *Your Brain on Porn*. Margate, Kent, UK: Commonwealth Publishing, 2017.

Yiannitsiotis, Constantine. *With Elder Porphyrios: A Spiritual Child Remembers*. Translated by Marina Robb. Milessi, Greece: The Transfiguration of the Savior, 2013.

Scripture Index

219

Subject Index

A

abstinence, from pornography, 34

abuse. *See* sexual abuse

acceptance, self-, 72, 117, 150, 191–92

acquisitive desire, 91

Adam and Eve, 93, 144, 145, 170

addiction, 49–50, 53, 76, 95, 105–7, 113–14, 149, 180

agape, 40

agnosia (unknowing), 128, 147–48

Alcoholics Anonymous (AA), 74n7, 106, 107n5. *See also* twelve-step programs

anger, 69, 90, 110–11, 110n9

animated porn, 27, 84

anonymity, 29

Anthony the Great, 158–59

anxiety, 67, 110–11

apophatic theology, 148, 148n5

Arendt, Hannah, 147

asceticism, 4–5, 115–16, 120–21, 163, 187–88, 207

assumptions, 141

Athanasius of Alexandria, 16

Augustine, 55, 186, 198, 203–4

avoidance (escapism), 28, 84–85, 111–12, 116–17

awareness, self-, 51–52, 89–90, 116–17, 120, 185, 190

B

Beausobre, Iulia de, 152–53, 153n10, 154

Bible, 138

black magic, 139

body: of death, 48–49, 105; unity with mind and spirit, 18–19

brain, 61–62, 83–84, 83n3, 112, 113–14

Breck, John, 41

Brown, Brené, 68n2

Bundy, Ted, 35n32

C

cam sites, 23n5, 24n8

canons, 189

celebrities, as icons, 135

certainty, 148

character formation, 17–18. *See also* neuroplasticity

chat, online sexualized, 23, 24n8

Weil, Simone, 152
Winnicott, Donald, 146,
   146n3
world. *See* creation

Y

Yiannitsiotis, Constantine, 144

Z

Zillman-Bryant experiments,
   33–34, 33n27, 39
Zinon (Theodore), Archimandrite,
   131, 133–34
Zosimas (saint), 97–98, 178, 179,
   181–82, 183, 184

About the Author

Andrew Williams works as a health care chaplain in both mental health and acute hospital contexts and is one of the teachers of a post-graduate course in psycho-spiritual care. He is also a counselor/psychotherapist with particular experience working with children and teens, domestic abuse, and issues relating to sexuality and intimacy. His interest in anthropology and the nature of interpersonal relationships led to his work on the Ancient Faith pastoral podcast "Finding the Freedom to Live in the Image of God" (FtFtL) during his time studying at Holy Cross Greek Orthodox School of Theology in Boston, where he graduated as valedictorian in 2010 with an MDiv. Also a graduate of Oxford University, sometime schoolteacher and musician, sometime resident of Russia, the USA, and France, he currently lives with his family in Oxford, England.

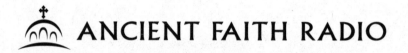